EXOTIC VIRAL DISEASES

1st Addendum

Severe Acute Respiratory Syndrome (SARS)

BERGER • CALISHER • KEYSTONE

2003
BC Decker Inc
Hamilton • London
www.bcdecker.com

Severe Acute Respiratory Syndrome* (SARS)

*Note: This chapter was written only 2 weeks into the initial outbreak of SARS in 2003. Clinical and epidemiologic data are therefore preliminary.

Agent: as yet unnamed coronavirus, family *Coronaviridae*

Reservoir: humans

Vector: none

Vehicle: respiratory secretions

Incubation period: 3d–5d (range 2d–10d)

Clinical hints:

cough	myalgia
fever	ongoing outbreak
headache	respiratory distress

Typical therapy: supportive, possibly ribavarin

Disease distribution:

China	Singapore
Hong Kong	Taiwan
Macao	Thailand
	Vietnam

Notes

In November 2002, a number of patients with signs of respiratory infection were reported in China. Subsequent cases were reported in other Asian countries and among persons who had recently visited Asia and returned to Europe, Australia, and North America. Preliminary studies suggest that the etiologic agent is a coronavirus. The pattern of disease acquisiton and

Exotic Viral Diseases
A Global Guide

Exotic Viral Diseases
A Global Guide

Stephen A. Berger, MD
Professor of Medicine
Tel Aviv University School of Medicine
Director of Medicine
Tel Aviv Medical Center
Tel Aviv, Israel

Charles H. Calisher, PhD
Professor of Microbiology,
Immuniology, and Pathology
Colorado State University
Fort Collins, Colorado

Jay S. Keystone, MD, MSc (CTM), FRCPC
Professor of Medicine
Center for Travel and Tropical Medicine
University of Toronto
Toronto, Ontario

2003
BC Decker Inc
Hamilton • London

WC
500
B47c
2003

BC Decker Inc
P.O. Box 620, L.C.D. 1
Hamilton, Ontario L8N 3K7
905-522-7017; 800-568-7281
Fax: 905-522-7839; 888-311-4987
E-mail: info@bcdecker.com
www.bcdecker.com

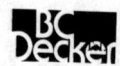

© 2003 BC Decker Inc

All rights reserved. No part of this publication may be reproduced, stored in a retrieval system, or transmitted, in any form or by an means, electronic, mechanical, photocopying, recording, or otherwise, without prior written permission from the publisher.

02 03 04 05/GSA/9 8 7 6 5 4 3 2 1

ISBN 1-55009-205-7
Printed in Spain

Sales and Distribution

United States
BC Decker Inc
P.O. Box 785
Lewiston, NY 14092-0785
Tel: 905-522-7017; 800-568-7281
Fax: 905-522-7839; 888-311-4987
E-mail: info@bcdecker.com
www.bcdecker.com

Canada
BC Decker Inc
20 Hughson Street South
P.O. Box 620, LCD 1
Hamilton, Ontario L8N 3K7
Tel: 905-522-7017; 800-568-7281
Fax: 905-522-7839; 888-311-4987
E-mail: info@bcdecker.com
www.bcdecker.com

Foreign Rights
John Scott & Company
International Publishers' Agency
P.O. Box 878
Kimberton, PA 19442
Tel: 610-827-1640
Fax: 610-827-1671
E-mail: jsco@voicenet.com

Japan
Igaku-Shoin Ltd.
Foreign Publications Department
3-24-17 Hongo
Bunkyo-ku, Tokyo, Japan 113-8719
Tel: 3 3817 5680
Fax: 3 3815 6776
E-mail: fd@igaku-shoin.co.jp

U.K., Europe, Scandinavia, Middle East
Elsevier Science
Customer Service Department
Foots Cray High Street
Sidcup, Kent
DA14 5HP, UK
Tel: 44 (0) 208 308 5760
Fax: 44 (0) 181 308 5702
E-mail: cservice@harcourt.com

Singapore, Malaysia, Thailand, Philippines, Indonesia, Vietnam, Pacific Rim, Korea
Elsevier Science Asia
583 Orchard Road
#09/01, Forum
Singapore 238884
Tel: 65-737-3593
Fax: 65-753-2145

Australia, New Zealand
Elsevier Science Australia
Customer Service Department
STM Division
Locked Bag 16
St. Peters, New South Wales, 2044
Australia
Tel: 61 02 9517-8999
Fax: 61 02 9517-2249
E-mail: stmp@harcourt.com.au
www.harcourt.com.au

Mexico and Central America
ETM SA de CV
Calle de Tula 59
Colonia Condesa
06140 Mexico DF, Mexico
Tel: 52-5-5553-6657
Fax: 52-5-5211-8468
E-mail: editoresdetextosmex@prodigy.net.mx

Argentina
CLM (Cuspide Libros Medicos)
Av. Córdoba 2067 – (1120)
Buenos Aires, Argentina
Tel: (5411) 4961-0042/(5411) 4964-0848
Fax: (5411) 4963-7988
E-mail: clm@cuspide.com

Brazil
Tecmedd
Av. Maurílio Biagi, 2850
City Ribeirão Preto – SP – CEP: 14021-000
Tel: 0800 992236
Fax: (16) 3993-9000
E-mail: tecmedd@tecmedd.com.br

Notice: The authors and publisher have made every effort to ensure that the patient care recommended herein, including choice of drugs and drug dosages, is in accord with the accepted standard and practice at the time of publication. However, since research and regulation constantly change clinical standards, the reader is urged to check the product information sheet included in the package of each drug, which includes recommended doses, warnings, and contraindications. This is particularly important with new or infrequently used drugs. Any treatment regimen, particularly one involving medication, involves inherent risk that must be weighed on a case-by-case basis against the benefits anticipated. The reader is cautioned that the purpose of this book is to inform and enlighten; the information contained herein is not intended as, and should not be employed, as a substitute for individual diagnosis and treatment.

spread suggests droplet infection, with health care personnel accounting for a large percentage of patients. Close contact with respiratory secretions appears to be the primary vehicle.

As of April 2, 2003, a total of 2,226 cases (78 fatal) were reported. Endemic or potentially endemic countries to date are China, Hong Kong, Macao, Singapore, Taiwan, Thailand, and Vietnam. Patients arriving from these countries were reported in Australia, Belgium, Canada, France, Germany, Ireland, Italy, Romania, Slovenia, Spain, Switzerland, the United Kingdom, and the United States; and secondary infection was acquired from patients arriving to Canada. Most patients have been previously healthy and in the age group 25 to 70 years.

Clinical presentation: The case definition for SARS consists of fever, cough, and respiratory difficulty, following exposure in an endemic country or to a patient suffering from the disease. Most patients report headache, sore throat, myalgia, and chills. Additional findings reported in some patitents include rhinorrhea, chest pain, diarrhea, vomiting, and confusion. Initial reports described isolated instances of "rash." Lymphocytopenia, neutropenia, thrombocytopenia, and elevations of creatine phosphokinase and hepatic transaminase levels are common. After 3 to 7 days, lower respiratory symptoms occur, particularly a dry, nonproductive cough, which may be accompanied by hypoxemia. Features of "atypical pneumonia" develop on the fourth to fifth days of illness. Ten to twenty percent of patients described to date have developed signs of adult respiratory distress syndrome. Chest roentgenograms reveal generalized interstitial or patchy infiltrates, with areas of consolidation in a few cases. The overall case-fatality rate is 3.7%, but can be as high as 50% among those who develop severe respiratory illness.

Specimens for diagnostic testing: respiratory secretions, serum, lung tissue

Patient isolation precautions: strict glove and mask precautions. Health care personnel and family members of cases appear to be at highest risk.

Suggested assays for virus detection: detection of viral RNA by PCR

Serodiagnosis: enzyme-linked immunosorbent assay test currently under development

Biosafety level required for working with the virus of SARS: not yet determined

Additional reading

Anon. Update: Outbreak of severe acute respiratory syndrome — worldwide, 2003. MMWR Morb Mortal Wkly Rep 2003;52;241–8.

Health Canada. Epidemiology, Clinical Presentation and Laboratory Investigation of Severe Acute Respiratory Syndrome (SARS) in Canada, March 2003. Available at: http://www.hc-sc.gc.ca/pphb-dgspsp/publicat/ccdr- (accessed March 31, 2003).

World Health Organization. Cumulative Number of Reported Cases (SARS). Available at: http://www.who.int/csr/sarscountry/2003_03_31/en (accessed March 31, 2003).

World Health Organization. Case Definitions for Surveillance of Severe Acute Respiratory Syndrome (SARS). Available at: http://www.who.int/csr/sars/casedefinition/en (accessed March 31, 2003).

Every Decker book is accompanied by a CD-ROM.

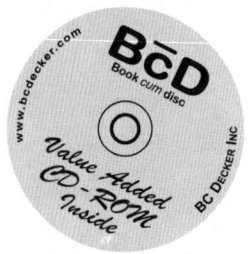

The disc appears in the front of each copy, in its own sealed jacket. Affixed to the front of the book will be a distinctive BcD sticker **"Book *cum* disc."**

The disc contains the complete text and illustrations of the book, in fully searchable PDF files. The book and disc are sold *only* as a package; neither is available independently, and no prices are available for the items individually.

BC Decker Inc is committed to providing high-quality electronic publications that complement traditional information and learning methods.

We trust you will find the book/CD package invaluable and invite your comments and suggestions.

Brian C. Decker
CEO and Publisher

CONTENTS

Preface xi
Acknowledgments xii

Introduction 1
Argentine hemorrhagic fever.............................. 22
Barmah Forest virus disease 26
Bolivian hemorrhagic fever............................... 31
Brazilian hemorrhagic fever 34
Bunyavirus infections (miscellaneous) 36
California serogroup virus infections 43
Chikungunya virus infection.............................. 48
Colorado tick fever 52
Cowpox disease 55
Crimean-Congo hemorrhagic fever 58
Dengue fever/dengue hemorrhagic fever 64
Eastern equine encephalitis.............................. 71
Ebola hemorrhagic fever.................................. 76
Group C viral fevers 80
Hantavirus infections (New World) 83
Hantavirus infections (Old World)........................ 89
Hendra disease 95
Herpes virus B infection 98
Ilheus and Bussuquara fevers 101
Japanese encephalitis 103
Kyasanur Forest disease 107
Lassa fever 110
Louping ill 114
Lymphocytic choriomeningitis 116
Marburg virus disease 119
Mayaro fever.. 122

- Monkeypox disease 125
- Murray Valley encephalitis 128
- New World sandfly fevers 132
- Nipah virus disease 134
- Old World sandfly fevers 137
- Omsk hemorrhagic fever 140
- O'nyong-nyong fever 143
- Orf virus disease 146
- Oropouche fever 148
- Powassan encephalitis 151
- Pseudocowpox disease 154
- Rift Valley fever 156
- Rocio encephalitis 160
- Ross River disease 162
- Sindbis fever 166
- Spondweni fever 170
- St. Louis encephalitis 173
- Tanapox virus disease 177
- Thogoto virus disease 179
- Tick-borne encephalitis (Central European) 182
- Tick-borne encephalitis (Russian spring-summer) 186
- Venezuelan equine encephalitis 189
- Venezuelan hemorrhagic fever 193
- Vesicular stomatitis 196
- Wesselsbron disease 199
- West Nile virus fever, West Nile virus encephalitis 202
- Western equine encephalitis 208
- Whitewater Arroyo virus infection 211
- Yellow fever 214
- Etiologic agents of exotic viral diseases 221

Appendix A: Sample collection, shipment, and testing ... 227
Appendix B: Diagnostic tests 230
Appendix C: Drugs and vaccines 235

Index.. *245*

Preface

No field in science evolves as rapidly as Clinical Virology. As you read these words, exotic human diseases are occurring all over the world. Each day heralds new outbreaks and epidemics by heretofore unfamiliar pathogens. Health care workers are confronted with exotic names like, "Ebola," "Hanta" and "West Nile" which until recent years were not even mentioned in standard medical texts. Just as new diseases appear, new disciplines evolve to confront these exotic illnesses: Travel Medicine, Emerging Infectious Diseases, and Geographic Medicine. Renewed interest in bio-terrorism has further underscored the significance of many of the viruses included in these pages.

Although a small number of texts have been written on the biology of Exotic Viral Agents, none have attempted to catalogue the practical clinical aspects of Exotic Viral Diseases. This book is specifically designed to summarize a vast body of clinical and epidemiological material on these conditions for the Heath Care Worker. In preparing the manuscript, the authors enjoyed considerable enthusiasm for the project; and a synergy and momentum which comes from sharing decades of experience in Virology, Infectious Diseases, and Tropical Medicine. As such, we would invite the reader to join in our enthusiasm for the subject, and trust that this text will fill an important niche in the clinician's arsenal.

Acknowledgments

To our families, who often found themselves speaking to our backs while we teased this book from the computer.

Steve

I want to thank Leonard Munstermann for the CD with the photos of the mosquitoes. To Steve Berger, for having gotten me roped into this in the first place. To Jay Keystone, for being one of the few people shorter than I am. To my parents, for something (I can't recall).

Charlie

I want to thank Charlie Calisher and Stephen Berger, without whom this book would have only been a dream . . . they did the bulk of the work and I rode in on their coat tails.

Jay

Introduction

There are about 100 generic viral diseases of humans (from Adenovirus to Zoster infections) of which more than half are included in this book as being due to infections by exotic viruses. We have defined exotic viruses as those that are geographically limited, rarely encountered, or rarely considered. As one might expect, what is exotic in one location may be commonplace in another. Japanese encephalitis, for example, is considered to be exotic in western countries, where it is rarely reported, but the disease is less exotic in Thailand, Japan, and other parts of Asia, despite that these countries may have well-developed universal immunization programs. In another respect, viral infections such as measles and polio, which were frequently encountered in the past and still occur occasionally, may be eliminated in the near future, and hence become exotic.

If exotic diseases are indeed rarely encountered in industrialized nations, it would be reasonable to ask, "Why bother writing this book at all?" The answer to the question has become abundantly clear in recent months. Viruses exotic to industrialized nations could find their way across oceans and borders with the help of humans, be it by intentional or non-intentional means. Nations have been known to be experimenting with germ warfare since the turn of the twentieth century. Bioterrorists could introduce a disease agent that is exotic to the place in which it is released, or they could release a hitherto controlled, long-eliminated, or eradicated agent, such as smallpox. Clinicians will inextricably find themselves on the front line of emergence of such problems, and this necessitates them to be well aware and educated. It is not so much that they must be able to conduct the laboratory tests themselves, but that they must be able to quickly and properly overview the disease sources and related references, and contact the proper authorities. Furthermore, in a world in which more than 500 million people cross international borders by aircraft every year, and where one can reach virtually any point on the globe within 36 hours, well within the incubation period for most exotic viral infections, clinicians are bound to encounter one or more exotic viruses within the course of their careers. When this happens, the obvious clinical question will be: "What viral infections can one acquire in location X, transmitted by vector Y, that look clinically like disease Z?"

This book has been designed to provide clinicians, travel medicine practitioners, geographic medicine specialists, infectious disease consultants, and medical microbiologists with a tool for assisting in the evaluation of a patient from a remote area or with an otherwise exotic disease. The reader will be able to consider a specific diagnosis on the basis of presenting symptoms, known exposure, and geographic location. In addition, this book is an ideal reference for teaching trainees in all areas of medicine, particularly medical microbiology and infectious diseases.

For those who are not versed in the standard terminology regarding the epidemiology of infectious disease, it is worth defining several basic terms that are crucial to the understanding of exotic viral disease transmission.

Vector: An arthropod or other living carrier that transports an infectious agent from an infected reservoir to a susceptible individual or immediate surroundings.

Vehicle: The mode of transmission for an infectious agent. This generally implies a passive and inanimate (ie, nonvector) mode.

Reservoir: Any animal, arthropod, plant, or substance in which an infectious agent normally lives and multiplies, on which it depends primarily for survival, and where it reproduces itself in such a manner that it can be transmitted to a susceptible host.

Dr. Steven Ostroff, deputy director of NCID (the National Center for Infectious Disease) at CDC in Atlanta, Georgia, once remarked, "Our global village provides global opportunities for the spread of infectious diseases." The recent introduction of West Nile virus into North America is a clear example of this new paradigm; intentionally-introduced anthrax in the United States is another. It is incumbent on infectious disease clinicians and medical microbiologists to be prepared to meet these new challenges. We trust that this monograph will help to inform students and colleagues, and to assist clinicians in their quest to provide excellent patient care in a global context. After all, any patient is potentially the first of an infectious disease outbreak, which threatens not only the patient but also the community at large.

Approach to the patient who may have an exotic viral disease

The assessment of a febrile patient who may be infected with an exotic virus begins with two important considerations:

1. Is this a medical emergency?
2. Is this patient a public health risk to health care providers or the community?

In the first instance, a rapid diagnosis is important in order to initiate potential life-saving therapy. Lassa fever virus and herpes virus B infections are two examples for which therapy should be initiated as soon as possible to reduce morbidity and mortality. In the second instance, the initiation of strict isolation procedures will be important to prevent spread of infection to hospital, laboratory, or clinic staff, and to the community. The African hemorrhagic fever viruses: Lassa, Marburg, and Ebola, are examples of the second category. Because some of the viruses outlined herein are **extremely dangerous**, we recommend that advice be sought from national or international experts when an exotic disease is suspected.

In order to make the above two assessments, it will be important for the clinician to determine whether or not the febrile patient may have an infection with an exotic virus. Assuming that the patient came from a tropical environment, the geographic, exposure, and clinical histories play significant roles in determining the likely risk. The travel history must include the countries visited, as well as whether the traveler had spent time in urban or rural areas. For example, many of the exotic viruses in this book are found only in rural areas; therefore, a history only of urban travel virtually rules out the possibility of such infections. Each of the diseases in this text is accompanied by a listing of "Disease distribution"; that is, countries which are known to be endemic or potentially endemic for the disease in question, or in which serosurveys and animal studies suggest recent presence of the disease.

The exact arrival and departure dates of travelers are critical in determining the minimal or maximal incubation period for infections being considered in the differential diagnosis. These dates must include arrival and departure times in rural areas as well as in urban centers. For example, individuals who departed from Nigeria are unlikely to be at risk for Lassa fever if they developed an illness more than 3 weeks after leaving a rural area, even if their departure from Nigeria was less than a week before the onset of their illness. In addition, since many of the infections discussed in this monograph are transmitted by arthropods, the season during which travel occurred might be an important determining factor as to whether or not a patient is at risk for infection. For example, Japanese encephalitis is transmitted throughout the year in tropical locations, but only during summer months in temperate zones.

Finally, it will be important for the clinician to take a careful immunization history, including the dates on which the vaccines were administered. Yellow fever and Japanese encephalitis can virtually be ruled out if a traveler was immunized appropriately, and was still within the known period of protection.

An exposure history is relevant to the consideration of an exotic viral disease. A history of a tick bite might suggest the diagnosis of infections such as Crimean-Congo hemorrhagic fever, Powassan encephalitis, or Kyasanur Forest disease. A history of mosquito bites, however, is often so inaccurate that it renders the question irrelevant and unnecessary. Unless the season dictates otherwise, one must assume the likelihood of a mosquito bite in endemic areas.

Close contact with rodents or other animals should raise the possibility of infections such as caused by herpes virus B, Lassa virus, Crimean-Congo hemorrhagic fever virus, Nipah virus, and hantaviruses. It is here that the occupational history (veterinarian, farmer, etc) may be crucial to determining a particular exposure. It will be important to know whether the patient has had close contact with infected or ill individuals, particularly in the setting of an outbreak of an infectious disease known to be transmitted from person-to-person. The most frequent consideration will be an exposure to an individual infected with an African hemorrhagic fever virus.

It would be helpful for the clinician to have some basic information of geographic medicine and a current knowledge of infectious disease outbreaks globally; the latter are available from electronic information networks such as Centers for Disease Control and Prevention (CDC), World Health Organization (WHO), Health Canada, ProMed, and GIDEON, among others.

Table 1 contains a list of key vectors, Table 2 is a list of virus transmission routes, and Table 3 is a list of reservoirs for the exotic viruses listed in this text.

Unfortunately, the clinical history may not be very helpful in establishing the diagnosis of an exotic viral infection. Many viral infections have similar features, and virtually all present with fever. The fever pattern itself is usually not very helpful although, occasionally, the presence of "saddle-back fever" can give a clue to the causative agent for the illness. Particular clinical syndromes, such as arthritis, rash, or encephalitis, can point the clinician to an appropriate differential diagnosis. Table 4 contains a list of clinical syndromes associated with particular exotic viral infections. However, the problem is that many of these exotic viral infections have a spectrum of diseases, ranging from a mild flu-like illness to severe symptoms, followed by death. Although it would not be difficult to make a diagnosis of a viral hemorrhagic fever in a returned traveler who has multiple bleeding sites and cutaneous hemorrhages, these findings do not usually occur until the second week of illness. The early stages of most exotic viral infections are nonspecific with fever, headache, and myalgia — symptoms similar to localized viral infections. Therefore, the consideration of an exotic viral infection begins with the presence of fever alone, and it becomes more specific with the clinical presentation associated with that fever.

The definitive diagnosis of an exotic viral infection is most often made through the use of acute and convalescent serology. In specific instances, viral isolation by culture or rapid diagnostic techniques such as reverse transcription-polymerase chain reaction (RT-PCR) are very helpful, but may not be readily available to the practicing clinician. Appendix A contains a brief review of the types of samples needed for laboratory diagnosis and the methods of shipment of those samples. Appendix B contains a brief review of diagnostic methods used to confirm suspected exotic viral infections.

Unfortunately, treatment of exotic viral infections is rather unsatisfactory, as there are only a few diseases for which drug therapy has been shown to be effective. However, for the infections that do respond to antiviral therapy, treatment may be life saving. The only two drugs that have been shown to be effective in the management of exotic viral infections are Acyclovir and Ribavirin. Appendix C contains a summary of these two agents. For further information, the reader is referred to the excellent publication prepared by the United States Pharmacopoeia Drug Information Service, *Health Information for the Health-care Professional*, published annually by Micromedex.

Even if treatment is unavailable, the potential public health impact may be an important consideration in the management of a dangerous exotic viral infection. Most industrialized countries have a contingency plan that lays out the steps to be followed in the event that a clinician or public health official is faced with an individual who may be infected with an exotic virus capable of spreading readily from person-to-person. Although the details of the approach are provided in these publications, it would be useful for the reader to know where to start should such an event occur.

Once an individual has been identified with a potentially contagious and dangerous exotic viral infection, such as an African hemorrhagic fever, isolation procedures, including use of gown, gloves, and mask, should be initiated. Any specimens that had been sent to the laboratory should be identified and held separately. It is noteworthy that there have been several well-documented patient deaths due to malaria, because appropriate investigations were put on hold when an exotic virus was suspected. In particular, where applicable, the diagnosis of malaria should be ruled out immediately under microbiologically secure conditions. Local public health officials should be informed as soon as possible, and if a public health risk is still deemed to be present, the public relations officer of the hospital or clinic should be notified. Unfortunately, once this process has been initiated, patient care may be jeopardized by health fears aroused in clinical care and laboratory staff, as well as by inappropriate media involvement.

For the most part, the prevention of exotic viral infections entails personal protection measures to prevent insect bites, avoidance of exposure to animals and ill persons, and other common sense precautions. In a few cases, notably yellow fever, Japanese encephalitis, and tick-borne encephalitis, excellent vaccines are available (see Appendix C). However, a reputable health care provider must administer these vaccines in sufficient time to ensure adequate protection prior to potential exposure.

Appendix B provides an outline of diagnostic tests that are recommended. Misplaced confidence in one's knowledge of, and resistance to, a potentially hazardous virus is a potentially fatal error. The nonimmune laboratory worker is no less resistant to infectious agents than are other individuals in the general population. Therefore, when considering whether and how to collect samples, conduct diagnostic assays, or ship specimens, the recommended level of safety and containment should be followed. Detailed recommendations are available from the US Centers for Disease Control and Prevention. Wherever two safety levels (one for handling tissues, another for manipulating viruses) have been recommended for a virus, the higher level is given.

Additional reading

Anon. Management of patients with suspected viral hemorrhagic fever. Morb Mort Wkly Rep 1998;37 Suppl 3:1–16.

Anon. Canadian contingency plan for viral hemorrhagic fevers and other related diseases. Can Commun Dis Rep 1997;23 Suppl 1:1–25.

US Centers for Disease Control and Prevention. Biosafety levels. Available at: http://www.cdc.gov/od/ohs/biosfty/bmbl4/bmbl4s7f.htm (accessed September 21, 2002).

Table 1 Vectors of Exotic Viruses

Vector	Virus transmitted
Mosquito	Barmah Forest virus
	Bunyavirus infections (miscellaneous)
	California encephalitis virus
	Chikungunya virus
	Dengue viruses
	Eastern equine encephalitis virus
	Group C viruses
	Ilheus virus
	Japanese encephalitis virus
	Mayaro virus
	Murray Valley encephalitis virus
	O'nyong-nyong virus
	Oropouche virus
	Rift Valley fever virus
	Rocio virus
	Ross River virus
	Sindbis virus
	Spondweni virus
	St. Louis encephalitis virus
	Venezuelan equine encephalitis virus
	Wesselsbron virus
	West Nile virus
	Western equine encephalitis virus
	Yellow fever virus
Tick	Colorado tick fever virus
	Crimean-Congo hemorrhagic fever virus
	Kyasanur Forest disease virus

(continued on next page)

Table 1 *(continued)*

	Louping ill virus
	Omsk hemorrhagic fever virus
	Powassan virus
	Thogoto virus
	Tick-borne encephalitis virus (Central European)
	Tick-borne encephalitis virus (Russian spring-summer)
Midge	Oropouche virus
Animal Bite or Oral Secretions	Hantaviruses
	Herpes virus B
	Lymphocytic choriomeningitis virus

Table 2 Routes of Viral Transmission

Animal Contact

Argentine hemorrhagic fever (Junin) virus
Bolivian hemorrhagic fever (Machupo) virus
Cowpox virus
Hantaviruses
Herpes virus B
Lassa virus
Marburg virus
Monkeypox virus
Orf virus
Pseudocowpox virus
Tanapox virus
Vesicular stomatitis viruses

Dairy Products

Louping ill virus
Powassan virus
Tick-borne encephalitis virus (Central European)
Tick-borne encephalitis virus (Russian spring-summer)

Droplet, Dust, or Aerosol

Argentine hemorrhagic fever (Junin) virus
Crimean-Congo hemorrhagic fever virus
Hantaviruses
Hendra virus
Lassa virus
Lymphocytic choriomeningitis virus
Nipah virus
Vesicular stomatitis viruses

Table 3 Natural Reservoirs of Exotic Viruses

Bat

Bunyaviruses (miscellaneous)
Ebola virus (possibly)
Group C viruses
Hantaviruses
Hendra virus
Kyasanur Forest disease virus
Marburg virus
Nipah virus
West Nile virus

Bird

Bunyaviruses (miscellaneous)
Crimean-Congo hemorrhagic fever virus
Eastern equine encephalitis virus
Hantaviruses
Ilheus virus
Japanese encephalitis virus
Kyasanur Forest disease virus
Louping ill virus
Mayaro virus
Murray Valley encephalitis virus
Rocio virus
Sindbis virus
St. Louis encephalitis virus
Thogoto virus
Tick-borne encephalitis virus (Central European)
West Nile virus
Western equine encephalitis virus

(continued on next page)

Table 3 *(continued)*

Cat

Cowpox virus
Hendra virus

Cattle

Bunyaviruses (miscellaneous)
Cowpox virus
Crimean-Congo hemorrhagic fever virus
Eastern equine encephalitis virus
Kyasanur Forest disease virus
Pseudocowpox virus
Rift Valley fever virus
Tick-borne encephalitis virus (Central European)
Tick-borne encephalitis virus (Russian spring-summer)
Vesicular stomatitis viruses
Wesselsbron virus

Deer

Louping ill virus
Orf virus

Horse

Bunyaviruses (miscellaneous)
Eastern equine encephalitis virus
Hendra virus
Venezuelan equine encephalitis virus
Vesicular stomatitis viruses
West Nile virus
Western equine encephalitis virus

Marsupial (including Macropods)

Barmah Forest virus
Bunyaviruses (miscellaneous)

(continued on next page)

Table 3 *(continued)*

Group C viruses
Ross River virus
Yellow fever virus

Swine

Eastern equine encephalitis virus
Japanese encephalitis virus
Nipah virus
Vesicular stomatitis viruses

Primate (nonhuman)

Chikungunya virus
Dengue viruses
Ebola virus
Herpes virus B
Kyasanur Forest disease virus
Lymphocytic choriomeningitis virus
Marburg virus
Mayaro virus
Monkeypox virus
Tanapox virus
Yellow fever virus

Lagomorph (Rabbit or Hare)

California serogroup viruses
Colorado tick fever virus
Crimean-Congo hemorrhagic fever virus
Tick-borne encephalitis virus (Russian spring-summer)

Rodent

Argentine hemorrhagic fever (Junin) virus
Bolivian hemorrhagic fever (Machupo) virus
Brazilian hemorrhagic fever (Sabia) virus

(continued on next page)

Table 3 *(continued)*

Bunyaviruses (miscellaneous)
California serogroup viruses
Colorado tick fever virus
Group C viruses
Hantaviruses
Hendra virus
Kyasanur Forest disease virus
Lassa virus
Louping ill virus
Lymphocytic choriomeningitis virus
Monkeypox virus
New World phleboviruses
Omsk hemorrhagic fever virus
Powassan virus
Ross River virus
Sandfly fever viruses
Tick-borne encephalitis virus (Central European)
Tick-borne encephalitis virus (Russian spring-summer)
Venezuelan equine encephalitis virus
Venezuelan hemorrhagic fever (Guanarito) virus
Whitewater Arroyo virus

Sheep

Bunyaviruses (miscellaneous)
Crimean-Congo hemorrhagic fever virus
Kyasanur Forest disease virus
Louping ill virus
Orf virus
Rift Valley fever virus
Thogoto virus
Wesselsbron virus

Table 4 Differential Diagnosis by Syndrome or Symptom Complex

Arthritis or Prominent Arthralgia

Barmah Forest virus disease
Chikungunya virus infection
Dengue fever/dengue hemorrhagic fever
Ilheus and Bussuquara fevers
Lymphocytic choriomeningitis*
Mayaro fever
New World sandfly fevers
O'nyong-nyong fever
Oropouche fever
Ross River disease
Sindbis fever
Wesselsbron disease
West Nile virus fever

Conjunctivitis or Photophobia

Argentine hemorrhagic fever
Bolivian hemorrhagic fever
Brazilian hemorrhagic fever
Bunyavirus infections (miscellaneous)
Chikungunya virus infection
Colorado tick fever
Crimean-Congo hemorrhagic fever
Group C viral fevers
Hantavirus infections (Old World)
Kyasanur Forest disease
Lassa fever
Louping ill
Lymphocytic choriomeningitis

(continued on next page)

Table 4 (continued)

Murray Valley encephalitis
New World sandfly fevers
Old World sandfly fevers
O'nyong-nyong fever
Oropouche fever
Rift Valley fever
Rocio encephalitis
St. Louis encephalitis
Venezuelan equine encephalitis
Vesicular stomatitis
West Nile virus fever
Yellow fever

Encephalitis or Meningitis

Argentine hemorrhagic fever
Bolivian hemorrhagic fever
Brazilian hemorrhagic fever
Bunyavirus infections (miscellaneous)*
California serogroup virus infections
Crimean-Congo hemorrhagic fever
Eastern equine encephalitis
Herpes virus B infection
Ilheus and Bussuquara fevers
Japanese encephalitis
Kyasanur Forest disease
Lassa fever
Louping ill
Lymphocytic choriomeningitis
Murray Valley encephalitis
Nipah virus disease
Oropouche fever*

(continued on next page)

Argentine hemorrhagic fever (AHF)

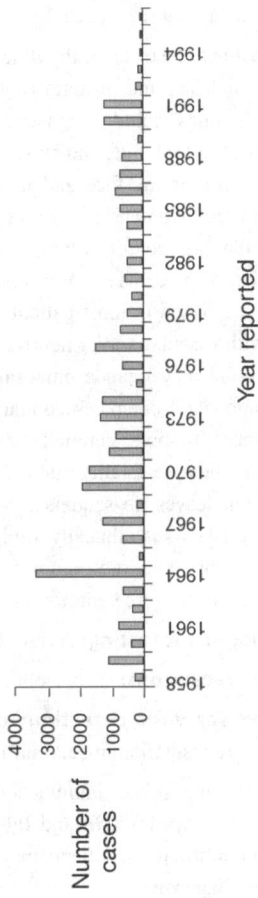

Figure 1 Argentine hemorrhagic fever in Argentina.

Nosocomial transmission has been documented. During the 1990s, 125 to 1,300 cases were reported yearly.

Clinical presentation: The onset of the illness is gradual, with progressive fever, malaise, and myalgia (notably in the lower back). Additional findings include epigastric pain, retro-orbital headache, dizziness, photophobia, and constipation. Conjunctival injection, erythema of the face and upper portion of the trunk, and orthostatic hypotension are common. Petechiae (notably in the axillae), generalized lymphadenopathy, and an enanthem consisting of petechiae and/or small vesicles on the palate and fauces are found in most patients. Patients become progressively ill with vascular and/or neurologic disease. Complications at this point may include mucosal bleeding, shock, pulmonary infiltration and edema, secondary bacterial infection, gait disturbances, tremors, cerebellar dysfunction, clonic seizures, and coma. The case-fatality rate is 30 to 40%. Convalescence is slow, but leaves no sequelae. Note that **Bolivian hemorrhagic fever (BHF)** is clinically similar to AHF; however, neurological signs are more common in AHF, whereas hemorrhagic diatheses are more common in BHF.

Specimens for diagnostic testing: serum, liver, spleen

Patient isolation precautions: strict isolation

Suggested assays for virus detection: detection of viral RNA by RT-PCR, virus isolation in cell cultures

Serodiagnosis: enzyme-linked immunosorbent assays and immunofluorescence assays for IgM and IgG antibodies, neutralization tests for confirmation; patients may not produce antibody useful for serodiagnosis

Biosafety level required for working with Junin virus: BSL-4

Additional reading

Buchmeier MJ, Bowen MD, Peters CJ. Arenaviridae: the viruses and their replication. In: Knipe DM, Howley PM, editors. Fields virology. Vol 2. 4th ed. Philadelphia: Lippincott Williams & Wilkins; 2001. p. 1635–68.

Carballal G, Videla CM, Merani MS. Epidemiology of Argentine hemorrhagic fever. Eur J Epidemiol 1988;4:259–74.

Enria DA, Maiztegui JI. Antiviral treatment of Argentine hemorrhagic fever. Antiviral Res 1994;23:23–31.

Harrison LH, Halsey NA, McKee KT Jr, et al. Clinical case definitions for Argentine hemorrhagic fever. Clin Infect Dis 1999;28:1091–4.

Maiztegui JI, McKee KT Jr, Barrera-Oro JG, et al. Protective efficacy of a live attenuated vaccine against Argentine hemorrhagic fever. J Infect Dis 1998;177:277–83.

Mills JN, Ellis BA, Childs JE, et al. Prevalence of infection with Junin virus in rodent populations in the epidemic area of Argentine hemorrhagic fever. Am J Trop Med Hyg 1994;51:554–62.

Mills JN, Ellis BA, McKee KT Jr, et al. A longitudinal study of Junin virus activity in the rodent reservoir of Argentine hemorrhagic fever. Am J Trop Med Hyg 1992;47:749–63.

http://www.cdc.gov/ncidod/dvrd/spb/mnpages/dispages/arena.htm (accessed September 21, 2002).

http://www.emedicine.com/emerg/topic887.htm (accessed September 21, 2002).

Barmah Forest virus disease (BFD)

Agent: Barmah Forest virus, family Togaviridae, genus *Alphavirus* (RNA) (a similar disease is caused by Ross River virus)

Reservoir: macropods (wallaby and kangaroo)

Vector: mosquito (*Aedes vigilax*, *Aedes camptorhynchus*, *Aedes normanensis*, *Culex* spp, *Coquillettidia* spp)

Vehicle: none

Incubation period: not established

Clinical hints:

arthralgia or arthritis (~ 60%)   less severe and protracted
fever (~ 91%)   than Ross River disease
rash

Typical therapy: symptomatic

Disease distribution: Australia (Figure 2)

Notes

Barmah Forest virus disease (BFD) is limited to Australia, and has been reported from all states, except Tasmania. Outbreaks often parallel those of Ross River disease.

The virus was first isolated from mosquitoes (*Culex annulirostris*) in the Barmah Forest, northern Victoria, in 1974. Human infection was subsequently reported along the south coast of New South Wales during the mid-1980s, in Queensland during 1988 to 1989, in the Northern Territory in 1992, and in southwestern Western Australia in 1993. A new focus was described in Gippsland, Victoria, during 1993 to 1994. In Queensland, 6.5% of healthy adults are seropositive.

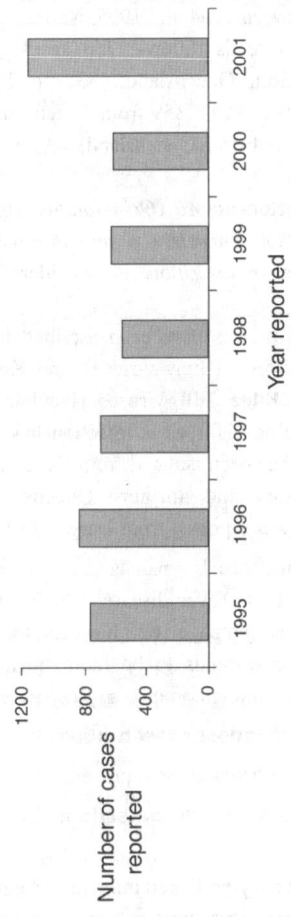

Figure 2 Barmah Forest virus disease in Australia.

More than 230 cases were reported from southeastern New South Wales between 1994 and 1995. Nationwide reports from 1995 to 2000 were as follows: 756 cases in 1995 (4.7 in 100,000; 456 from Queensland), 837 in 1996 (576 from Queensland), 704 in 1997 (359 from Queensland), 558 in 1998 (3.0 in 100,000; 354 from Queensland), 634 in 1999, and 1,162 in 2000.

The disease vectors are *Ae.* (*Ochlerotatus*) *vigilax*, *Ae. camptorhynchus*, *Ae. normanensis*, *Cx. annulirostris*, and *Coquillettidia* spp. *Aedes notoscriptus* is considered an additional potential vector.

Similar local illnesses have been ascribed to **Trubanaman** and **Gan Gan** viruses (Bunyaviridae), and **Kokobera**, **Alfuy**, **Stratford**, and **Edge Hill** viruses (Flaviviridae). A single human case of Edge Hill virus infection has been described. Kokobera virus has been isolated from *Cx. annulirostris* in the Northern Territory and northern Queensland. A case of Kokobera fever was reported from Darwin in 1998.

Clinical presentation: Barmah Forest virus disease is clinically similar to Ross River disease, which will be discussed later in this manual (on page 162); however, the rash of Barmah Forest virus disease tends to be more florid and vesicular, whereas arthritis is more common in Ross River disease

Specimens for diagnostic testing: serum

Patient isolation precautions: prevent access by mosquitoes

Suggested assays for virus detection: virus isolation in cell cultures

Serodiagnosis: enzyme-linked immunosorbent assays for IgM and IgG antibodies, neutralization tests for confirmation; cross-reactivity with Ross River virus can cause confusion

Biosafety level required for working with Barmah Forest virus: BSL-2

Additional reading

Anon. Barmah Forest virus [editorial]. Lancet 1991;337:948–9.

Doggett SL, Russell RC, Clancy J, et al. Barmah Forest virus epidemic on the south coast of New South Wales, Australia, 1994–1995: viruses, vectors, human cases, and environmental factors. J Med Entomol 1999;36:861–8.

Flexman JP, Smith DW, Mackenzie JS, et al. A comparison of the diseases caused by Ross River virus and Barmah Forest virus. Med J Aust 1998;169:159–63.

Griffin DE. Alphaviruses. In: Knipe DM, Howley PM, editors. Fields virology. Vol 1. 4th ed. Philadelphia: Lippincott Williams & Wilkins; 2001. p. 917–62.

Lindsay M, Johansen C, Broom AK, et al. Emergence of Barmah Forest virus in Western Australia. Emerg Infect Dis 1995;1:22–6.

Mackenzie JS, Broom AK, Hall RA, et al. Arboviruses in the Australian region, 1990 to 1998. Commun Dis Intell 1998;22:93–100.

Mackenzie JS, Lindsay MD, Coelen RJ, et al. Arboviruses causing human disease in the Australasian zoogeographic region. Arch Virol 1994;136:447–67.

Mackenzie JS, Smith DW. Mosquito-borne viruses and epidemic polyarthritis. Med J Aust 1996;164:90–3.

Nash P, Harrington T. Acute Barmah Forest polyarthritis. Aust N Z J Med 1991;21:737–8.

Schlesinger S, Schlesinger MJ. Togaviridae: the viruses and their replication. In: Knipe DM, Howley PM, editors. Fields virology. Vol. 1. 4th ed. Philadelphia: Lippincott Williams & Wilkins; 2001. p. 895–916.

http://www.arbovirus.health.nsw.gov.au/arbovirus/viruses/rossriverbarmahforest.htm (accessed September 21, 2002).
http://medicineau.net.au/clinical/medicine/medicine3.html (accessed September 21, 2002).

Bolivian hemorrhagic fever (BHF)
(Machupo hemorrhagic fever)

Agent: Machupo virus, family Arenaviridae, genus *Arenavirus* (RNA), Tacaribe complex

Reservoir: rodent (*Calomys callosus*)

Vector: none

Vehicle: food, water, excreta, direct patient contact

Incubation period: 5 d–19 d

Clinical hints:

agricultural setting	neurological findings
fever	petechiae
leukopenia	relative bradycardia
lymphadenopathy	spring and summer
myalgia	thrombocytopenia

Typical therapy: strict isolation; specific immune plasma; suggest Ribavirin 2.0 g IV, then 1.0 g IV q6h × 4 d, then 0.5 g IV q8h × 6 d

Disease distribution: Bolivia

Considered a potential bioterrorism weapon.

Notes

Bolivian hemorrhagic fever was first identified in 1959 as a sporadic hemorrhagic illness in rural areas of Beni Department, Bolivia.

The disease is most common during April to July, in the upper savanna region of eastern Bolivia (Beni). Eight cases were reported in 1999 (5 in Santa Cruz, 3 in Tarija), and 18 in 2000.

Principal exposure occurs through rodents (*C. callosus*) which enter homes in this region. Nosocomial and person-to-person spread have been documented. Infection of *C. callosus* results in asymptomatic viral shedding in saliva, urine, and feces; 50% of experimentally infected *C. callosus* are chronically viremic and shed virus in their bodily excreta or secretions. Although the infectious dose of Machupo virus in humans is unknown, exposed persons may become infected by inhaling virus in aerosolized secretions or excreta of infected rodents, ingestion of food contaminated with rodent excreta, or by direct contact of excreta with abraded skin or oropharyngeal mucous membranes. Reports of person-to-person transmission are uncommon. Hospital contact with a patient has resulted in person-to-person spread of Machupo virus to nursing and pathology laboratory staff. In 1994, the fatal secondary infection of six family members in Magdalena from a single naturally acquired infection further suggested the potential for person-to-person transmission.

Clinical presentation: Early clinical manifestations consist of nonspecific signs and symptoms including fever, headache, fatigue, myalgia, and arthralgia. Within 7 days, patients may hemorrhage from the oral and nasal mucosa and from the bronchopulmonary, gastrointestinal, and genitourinary tracts.

Specimens for diagnostic testing: serum, liver, spleen

Patient isolation precautions: strict isolation

Suggested assays for virus detection: detection of viral RNA by RT-PCR

Serodiagnosis: enzyme-linked immunosorbent assays for IgM and IgG antibodies, neutralization tests for confirmation

Biosafety level required for working with Machupo virus: BSL-4

Additional reading

Anon. Bolivian hemorrhagic fever. JAMA 1967;200:716–7.

Anon. From the Centers for Disease Control and Prevention. Bolivian hemorrhagic fever - El Beni Department, Bolivia, 1994. JAMA 1995;273:194–6.

Buchmeier MJ, Bowen MD, Peters CJ. Arenaviridae: the viruses and their replication, In: Knipe DM, Howley PM, editors. Fields virology. Vol. 2. 4th ed. Philadelphia: Lippincott Williams & Wilkins; 2001. p. 1635–68.

Kilgore PE, Ksiazek TG, Rollin PE, et al. Treatment of Bolivian hemorrhagic fever with intravenous ribavirin. Clin Infect Dis 1997;24:718–22.

Kilgore PE, Peters CJ, Mills JN, et al. Prospects for the control of Bolivian hemorrhagic fever [editorial]. Emerg Infect Dis 1995;1:97–100.

Stinebaugh BJ, Schloeder FX, Johnson KM, et al. Bolivian hemorrhagic fever. A report of four cases. Am J Med 1966;40:217–30.

http://www.cdc.gov/ncidod/dvrd/spb/mnpages/dispages/arena.htm (accessed September 21, 2002).

http://www.emedicine.com/emerg/topic887.htm (accessed September 21, 2002).

Brazilian hemorrhagic fever
(Sabia)

Agent: Sabia virus, family Arenaviridae, genus *Arenavirus* (RNA), Tacaribe complex

Reservoir: rodent (presumed)

Vector: none

Vehicle: excreta

Incubation period: 7 d (precise data lacking)

Clinical hints:

azotemia	myalgia
coma	neutropenia
fever	pharyngeal injection
gastrointestinal hemorrhage	seizures
headache	

Typical therapy: strict isolation; no therapy proven; suggest Ribavirin 2.0 g IV, then 1.0 g IV q6h × 4 d, then 0.5 g IV q8h × 6 d

Disease distribution: Brazil

Considered a potential bioterrorism weapon.

Notes

To date, only three cases of Sabia virus infection have been described, one of which was fatal; two of these cases were acquired in laboratories.

The first case was reported in Sao Paulo, Brazil in 1990. Infection was thought to have originated in a community called Sabia.

Clinical presentation: Clinically, Sabia is reminiscent of Argentine hemorrhagic fever, but natural infection is limited to Brazil.

Specimens for diagnostic testing: serum, liver, spleen

Patient isolation precautions: strict isolation

Suggested assays for virus detection: detection of viral RNA by RT-PCR

Serodiagnosis: enzyme-linked immunosorbent assays for IgM and IgG antibodies, neutralization tests for confirmation

Biosafety level required for working with Sabia virus: BSL-4

Additional reading

Anon. *Arenavirus* infection — Connecticut, 1994. MMWR Morb Mort Wkly Rep 1994;43:635–6.

Armstrong LR, Dembry LM, Rainey PM, et al. Management of a Sabia virus-infected patient in a US hospital. Infect Control Hosp Epidemiol 1999;20:176–82.

Barry M, Russi M, Armstrong L, et al. Brief report: treatment of a laboratory-acquired Sabia virus infection. N Engl J Med 1995;333:294–6.

Bowen MD, Peters CJ, Nichol ST. The phylogeny of New World (Tacaribe complex) arenaviruses. Virology 1996;219:285–90.

Buchmeier MJ, Bowen MD, Peters CJ. Arenaviridae: the viruses and their replication. In: Knipe DM, Howley PM, editors. Fields virology. Vol 2. 4th ed. Philadelphia: Lippincott Williams & Wilkins; 2001. p. 1635–68.

Coimbra TLM, Nassar ES, Burattini MN, et al. New arenavirus isolated in Brazil. Lancet 1994;343:391–2.

http://www.cdc.gov/ncidod/dvrd/spb/mnpages/dispages/arena.htm (accessed September 21, 2002).

http://www.emedicine.com/emerg/topic887.htm (accessed September 21, 2002).

Bunyavirus infections (miscellaneous)

Agent: any of more than 30 viruses belonging to the family Bunyaviridae, genus *Orthobunyavirus* (RNA)

Reservoir: rats, birds, marsupials, chipmunks, cattle, sheep, horses, bats

Vector: mosquito (exception: Shuni is transmitted by culicoid flies; Wanowrie, Bhanja, and Tamdy by ticks)

Vehicle: none

Incubation period: 3 d–12 d

Clinical hints:

abrupt onset of chills	myalgia
arthralgia	photophobia
cough	rash
diarrhea	vomiting
headache	2 to 7 day illness

Note: meningitis or myocarditis may occur with Bwamba virus

Typical therapy:

Disease distribution:

Angola	Cameroon
Argentina	Cape Verde
Belize	Central African Republic
Benin	Chad
Bolivia	Colombia
Botswana	Comoros
Brazil	Costa Rica
Bulgaria	Czechoslovakia (former)
Burkina Faso	Democratic Republic of
Burundi	Congo

- Djibouti
- Ecuador
- Egypt
- El Salvador
- Equatorial Guinea
- Ethiopia
- French Guiana
- Gabon
- Gambia
- Ghana
- Guatemala
- Guinea
- Guinea-Bissau
- Guyana
- Honduras
- India
- Italy
- Ivory Coast
- Kenya
- Lesotho
- Liberia
- Madagascar
- Malawi
- Mali
- Mexico
- Mozambique
- Namibia
- Nicaragua
- Niger
- Nigeria
- Pakistan
- Panama
- Paraguay
- Peru
- Portugal
- Reunion
- Romania
- Russia (former Soviet Union)
- Rwanda
- Sao Tome & Principe
- Senegal
- Sierra Leone
- Somalia
- South Africa
- Spain
- Sri Lanka
- Sudan
- Suriname
- Swaziland
- Tanzania
- Togo
- Trinidad & Tobago
- Uganda
- United States
- Uruguay
- Venezuela
- Yugoslavia (former)
- Zambia
- Zimbabwe

Notes

This group includes more than 30 viruses that cause human illness in the Americas and Africa. **Group C**, **phleboviruses**, **California serogroup**, and **Oropouche** viruses are discussed elsewhere in this manual. As a group, these are the most common mosquito-borne viruses in the world.

Most cause sporadic disease among persons living at the forest edge and engaged in outdoor activities, including military personnel. Outbreaks occasionally occur.

Bhanja virus is a tick-borne virus reported in India, Cameroon, Egypt, Bulgaria, Spain, Kenya, Italy, Portugal, Romania, Croatia, and the former Czechoslovakia. Signs range from a mild febrile illness to meningoencephalitis.

Bunyamwera virus is the ninth most common arthropod-borne virus in Africa. The principal vector is *Aedes (Neomelanoconion) circumluteolus*. Additional vectors include *Aedes pembaensis*, *Culex* spp, *Mansonia africana*, and *Mansonia uniformis*.

Garissa virus, a reassortant of **Bunyamwera** virus and an as yet unidentified member of this serogroup, was detected in patients in Kenya and Somalia during an outbreak of Rift Valley fever. Signs and symptoms in these patients mimicked those of Rift Valley fever.

Germiston, **Bwamba**, and **Ilesha** viruses are found in Africa. The principal vector for Germiston is *Culex (Eumelanomyia) rubinotus*. Additional vectors include *Ae. circumluteolus*, *Anopheles arabiensis*, and *Anopheles funestus*. *Culex theileri* has also been implicated. Ilesha virus is transmitted by *Anopheles gambiae* and *M. uniformis*. Bwamba virus is transmitted by *An. funestus* and *An. gambiae*.

Ngari virus is a mosquito-borne virus implicated in cases of meningoencephalitis in Senegal and Madagascar.

Tamdy virus has been associated with human infection in Central Asia, Kazakhstan, and Transcaucasia. Clinical features are nonspecific. The vector is *Hyalomma asiaticum*.

Pongola virus is mosquito-borne and has been associated with cases of arthritis. It is found in Kenya and Uganda.

Wanowrie is a tick-borne virus found in India and Sri Lanka, and is characterized by meningoencephalitis or hemorrhagic fever. The vector is *Hyalomma marginatum isaaci*.

Wyeomyia virus is found in South America, and may be transmitted by mosquitoes of at least 23 species, including species of *Aedes*, *Anopheles*, *Coquillettidia*, *Culex*, *Haemagogous*, *Limatus*, *Psorophora*, *Trichoprosopon*, and *Wyeomyia*.

Tensaw virus is found in North America. The principal vector is *Anopheles crucians*. Additional vectors include *Anopheles punctipennis*, *Anopheles quadrimaculatus*, *Aedes atlanticus*, *Aedes infirmatus*, *Aedes mitchellae*, *Coquillettidia perturbans*, *Culex nigripalpus*, and *Culex salinarius*.

Batai (= **Calovo**, **Lumbo**) virus was originally found in Asia and Europe. Antibody to Calovo virus was found among wild animals in the Czech Republic, Slovakia, Austria, Romania, the former Yugoslavia, Poland, and the former Soviet Union. Antibody to **Lumbo** virus was found among animals in Mozambique, Sri Lanka, and the former Soviet Union.

Fort Sherman, **Tacaiuma**, **Guama**, and **Catu** viruses occur in South America, whereas Cache Valley virus occurs in North America. Most of these viruses cause uncomplicated febrile illnesses but **Cache Valley** virus has been associated with abortion and teratology in animals and with human congenital anomalies and encephalitis.

Other viruses in this group, such as **Nyando** and **Shokwe** viruses, have been associated with febrile human illnesses in Africa.

Northway virus was first isolated from *Aedes* mosquitoes in 1971. Antibodies to this virus were found in 4 to 14% of Native Americans and Forest Service workers in Alaska in the 1980s. Two to 40 percent of cattle in many American states are seropositive to Northway, Cache Valley, and Tensaw viruses.

Clinical presentation: chills, fever, headache

Specimens for diagnostic testing: serum

Patient isolation precautions: prevent access by mosquitoes

Suggested assays for virus detection: virus isolation in cell cultures, detection of viral RNA by RT-PCR

Serodiagnosis: enzyme-linked immunosorbent assays for IgM and IgG antibodies, neutralization tests for confirmation

Biosafety level required for working with these viruses: depends on the virus; most are BSL-2, but others have been placed at BSL-3 because of insufficient experiences

Additional reading

Calisher CH, Coimbra TL, de S Lopez O, et al. Identification of new Guama and Group C serogroup bunyaviruses and an ungrouped virus from Southern Brazil. Am J Trop Med Hyg 1983;32:424–31.

Calisher CH, Lazuick JS, Lieb S, et al. Human infections with Tensaw virus in south Florida: evidence that Tensaw virus subtypes stimulate the production of antibodies reactive with closely related Bunyamwera serogroup viruses. Am J Trop Med Hyg 1988;39:117–22.

Calisher CH, Sever JL. Are North American Bunyamwera serogroup viruses etiologic agents of human congenital defects of the central nervous system? Emerg Infect Dis 1995;4:147–51.

Campbell GL, Hardy JL, Eldridge BF, Reeves WC. Isolation of Northway serotype and other Bunyamwera serogroup bunyaviruses from California and Oregon mosquitoes, 1969–1985. Am J Trop Med Hyg 1991;44:581–8.

Darwish MA, Hoogstraal H, Roberts TJ, et al. A seroepidemiological survey for Bunyaviridae and certain other arboviruses in Pakistan. Trans R Soc Trop Med Hyg 1983;77: 446–50.

Filipe AR, Calisher CH, Lazuick J. Antibodies to Congo-Crimean haemorrhagic fever, Dhori, Thogoto and Bhanja viruses in southern Portugal. Acta Virol 1985;29:324–8.

Gonzalez MT, Filipe AR. Antibodies to arboviruses in northwestern Spain. Am J Trop Med Hyg 1977;26:792–7.

Gordon SW, Tammariello RF, Linthicum KL, et al. Arbovirus isolations from mosquitoes collected during 1988 in the Senegal River basin. Am J Trop Med Hyg 1992;47:742–8.

Hubalek Z, Mittermayer T, Halouzka J, Cerny V. Isolation of "exotic" Bhanja virus (Bunyaviridae) from ticks in the temperate zone. Arch Virol 1988;101:191–7.

Johnson BK, Chanas AC, Squires EJ, et al. The isolation of a Bwamba virus variant from man in Western Kenya. J Med Virol 1978;2:15–20.

Johnson BK, Shockley P, Chanas AC, et al. Arbovirus isolations from mosquitoes: Kano Plain, Kenya. Trans R Soc Trop Med Hyg 1977;71:518–21.

Kalunda M, Lwanga-Ssozi C, Lule M, Mukuye A. Isolation of Chikungunya and Pongola viruses from patients in Uganda [letter]. Trans R Soc Trop Med Hyg 1985;79:567.

Lundstrom JO. Mosquito-borne viruses in western Europe: a review. J Vector Ecol 1999;24:1–39.

Lvov DK, Sidorova GA, Gromashevsky VL, et al. Virus "Tamdy" — a new arbovirus, isolated in the Uzbek S.S.R. and Turkmen S.S.R. from ticks *Hyalomma asiaticum asiaticum* Schulee and Schlottke, 1929, and *Hyalomma plumbeum plumbeum* Panzer, 1796. Arch Virol 1976;51:15–21.

Moore DL, Causey OR, Carey DE, et al. Arthropod-borne viral infections of man in Nigeria, 1964–1970. Ann Trop Med Parasitol 1975;69:49–64.

Morvan JM, Digoutte JP, Marsan P, Roux J-F. Ilesha virus: a new aetiological agent of haemorrhagic fever in Madagascar. Trans R Soc Trop Med Hyg 1994;88:205.

Nichol ST. Bunyaviruses. In: Knipe DM, Howley PM, editors. Fields virology. Vol 2. 4th ed. Philadelphia: Lippincott Williams & Wilkins; 2001. p. 1603–33.

Schmaljohn CS, Hooper JW. Bunyaviridae: the viruses and their replication. In: Knipe DM, Howley PM, editors. Fields virology. Vol 2. 4th ed. Philadelphia: Lippincott Williams & Wilkins; 2001. p. 1581–602.

Singh A, Padbidri VS. A retrospective serological survey of humans in India for Wanowrie virus. J Commun Dis 1998;30:89–92.

Tomori O, Monath TP, Lee V, et al. Bwamba virus infection: a sero-survey of vetebrates in five ecological zones in Nigeria. Trans R Soc Trop Med Hyg 1974;68:461–5.

van Tongeren H. Occurrence of arboviruses belonging to the C-, Bunyamwera and Guama groups, and of Oropouche, Junin, Tacaiuma and Kwatta viruses in man in the province of Brokopondo, Surinam: a serological survey. Trop Geogr Med 1967;19:309–25.

Walters LL, Tirrell SJ, Shope RE. Seroepidemiology of California and Bunyamwera serogroup (Bunyaviridae) virus infections in native populations of Alaska. Am J Trop Med Hyg 1999;60:806–21.

California serogroup virus infections

Agent: certain viruses of the family Bunyaviridae, genus *Orthobunyavirus* (RNA), California serogroup

Reservoir: chipmunk, squirrel, rodent, fox, rabbit

Vector: mosquito (*Ochlerotatus* [formerly *Aedes*] *triseriatus*, *Anopheles* spp, *Culex* spp, *Psorophora* spp)

Vehicle: none

Incubation period: 5 d–15 d

Clinical hints:

late summer flu-like illness	polymorphonuclear
meningitis or encephalitis	leucocytosis
paralysis common	seizures
	wooded areas

Typical therapy: symptomatic

Disease distribution:

Canada	Russia
China	Sweden
Czechoslovakia	United States
Finland	Yugoslavia (former)
Panama	

Notes

This group consists of viruses associated primarily with mild flu-like illness (Inkoo, Tahyna, Guaroa) or encephalitis (La Crosse, California encephalitis, Jamestown Canyon, and snow-shoe hare viruses).

La Crosse encephalitis accounts for most cases of California encephalitis in the United States, and is the most important cause of pediatric arboviral encephalitis there. Severe disease is largely restricted to children below the age of 15 years, with a male:female ratio in excess of 2:1. Disease is most common in areas of hardwood forests and woodlots, the primary habitat of the principal vector (Figure 3). The geographic range of this virus appears to be expanding, possibly due to its adaptation to the recent US invader, *Aedes albopictus*.

The principal vectors of these viruses in the United States are *Oc. triseriatus*, *Aedes dorsalis*, and *Aedes melanimon*. Additional vectors include *Aedes vexans*, *Aedes nigromaculis*, *Ae. albopictus*, *Anopheles pseudopunctipennis*, *Culex tarsalis*, *Culiseta inornata*, and *Psorophora* spp. The vector is infected for life, and the virus is transmitted transovarially.

The principal vector for La Crosse virus is *Oc. triseriatus*. Additional vectors include *Aedes canadensis* and *Aedes communis*.

Trivittatus virus may be a cause of self-limited febrile infections in the central and eastern United States.

Several instances of neurological infection in Florida have been ascribed to **Keystone** virus.

Snowshoe hare virus, a variety of La Crosse virus, has been associated with rare, but severe, neurological infections in Canada, China, and the United States.

Inkoo virus is transmitted by *Ae. communis* and *Aedes punctor*.

Tahyna virus is associated with respiratory infection in the Czech Republic and Slovakia. In Africa, the agent is transmitted by *Aedes pembaensis*. The principal European vector is *Ae. vexans*, with additional transmission by *Aedes cantans*, *Aedes caspius*, *Aedes cinereus*, *Anopheles hyrcanus*, *Anopheles maculipennis*, *Culex modestus*, *Culex pipiens*, and *Culiseta annulata*.

Clinical presentation: Infection of humans by California serogroup viruses is usually subclinical, or limited to a mild

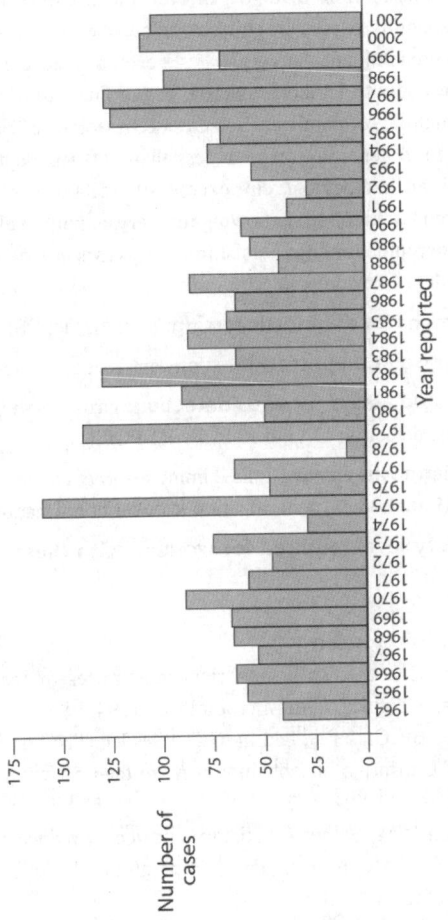

Figure 3 California serogroup encephalitis in the United States.

febrile illness. More than 90% of overt La Crosse virus meningoencephalitis occurs in children below the age of 15 years, with a predominance among males. Fever, headache, and vomiting progress to lethargy, aphasia, incoordination, focal motor abnormalities, or paralysis. Seizures occur in 50% of cases. The spinal fluid generally contains less than 100 leukocytes/mm^3. Peripheral leukocytosis in excess of 15,000 white blood cells/mm^3 is common. Following recovery, abnormal electroencephalographic findings persist for 1 to 5 years in 75% of cases, and epilepsy develops in 10%.

Specimens for diagnostic testing: brain tissue, CSF, serum

Patient isolation precautions: prevent access by mosquitoes

Suggested assays for virus detection: virus isolation in cell cultures, detection of viral RNA by RT-PCR

Serodiagnosis: enzyme-linked immunosorbent assays for IgM and IgG antibodies, neutralization tests for confirmation

Biosafety level required for working with these viruses: BSL-2

Additional reading

Calisher CH. Medically important arboviruses of the United States and Canada. Clin Microbiol Rev 1994;7:89–116.

Eldridge BF, Glaser C, Pedrin RE, Chiles RE. The first reported case of California encephalitis in more than 50 years. Emerg Infect Dis 2001;7:451–2.

Hammon WM, Sather G. History and recent reappearance of viruses in the California encephalitis group. Am J Trop Med Hyg 1966;15:199–204.

Jones TF, Craig AS, Nasci RS, et al. Newly recognized focus of La Crosse encephalitis in Tennessee. Clin Infect Dis 1999;28: 93–7.

Kitron U, Michael J, Swanson J, Haramis L. Spatial analysis of the distribution of La Crosse encephalitis in Illinois, using a geographic information system and local and global spatial statistics. Am J Trop Med Hyg 1997;57:469–75.

Nichol ST. Bunyaviruses. In: Knipe DM, Howley PM, editors. Fields virology. Vol 2. 4th ed. Philadelphia: Lippincott Williams & Wilkins; 2001. p. 1603–33.

Niklasson B, Vene S. Vector-borne viral diseases in Sweden — a short review. Arch Virol (Suppl) 1996;11:49–55.

Schmaljohn CS, Hooper JW. Bunyaviridae: the viruses and their replication. In: Knipe DM, Howley PM, editors. Fields virology. Vol 2. 4th ed. Philadelphia: Lippincott Williams & Wilkins; 2001. p. 1581–602.

Traavik T, Mehl R, Wiger R. California encephalitis group viruses isolated from mosquitoes collected in Southern and Arctic Norway. Acta Pathol Microbiol Scand 1978;86B:335–41.

http://www.cdc.gov/ncidod/dvbid/arbor/index.htm (accessed September 21, 2002).

http://www.cdc.gov/ncidod/diseases/list_mosquitoborne.htm (accessed September 21, 2002).

Chikungunya virus infection

Agent: Chikungunya virus, family Togaviridae, genus *Alphavirus* (RNA), related to Semliki Forest and Me Tri viruses, found in Africa and Asia

Reservoir: primate

Vector: mosquito (*Aedes aegypti*; *Aedes furcifer-taylori* group in Africa)

Vehicle: none

Incubation period: 2 d–12 d

Clinical hints:

abrupt fever	myalgia
leukopenia	prominent bilateral joint pain
maculopapular rash	pruritis

Typical therapy: symptomatic

Disease distribution:

Cambodia	Philippines
China	Saudi Arabia
Democratic Republic of Congo	Senegal
Guam	South Africa
India	Sri Lanka
Indonesia	Tanzania
Malaysia	Thailand
Myanmar	Uganda
Nigeria	Vietnam
Papua New Guinea	Zimbabwe

Notes

Chikungunya means "that which bends up" in the Makonde language of Newala Province, Tanzania. The virus was first isolated from humans during an outbreak in 1952 to 1953. A second outbreak occurred in South Africa in 1956.

Outbreaks are most common during the rainy season; epidemics lasting up to 6 years have been described in Asia.

A related alphavirus, Semliki Forest virus, causes a similar disease, and is occasionally implicated as an agent of febrile illness in Africa.

The principal African vector of chikungunya virus is *Aedes aegypti*. Additional vectors include *Aedes (Diceromyia) furcifer*, *Aedes (Stegomyia) africanus*, *Coquillettidia fuscopennata*, *Culex quinquefasciatus*, *Mansonia africana*, and *Mansonia uniformis*.

The principal Southeast Asian vector is *Ae. aegypti*. Additional vectors include *Aedes albopictus*, *Culex gelidus*, *Culex quinquefasciatus*, and *Culex tritaeniorhyncus*.

The vectors of Semliki Forest virus are *Aedes (Aedimorphus) abnormalis* group, *Aedes argenteopunctatus*, *Aedes denatus*, *Aedes (Neomelaniconion) palpalis*, *Aedes (Cellia) funestus*, and *Eretmapodites grahamii*.

Me Tri virus has been implicated as an agent of encephalitis among children in Vietnam.

Clinical presentation: The fever of Chikungunya is characterized by a rapid rise in temperature to as high as 40°C, often accompanied by rigors, myalgia, headache, photophobia, retro-orbital pain, sore throat with objective signs of pharyngitis, nausea, and vomiting. Fever may abate after a few days, only to recrudesce ("saddle-back" fever curve). Polyarthralgia favors small joints and sites of previous injury, and is most intense on arising. Joints may swell, but without significant fluid accumulation. These symptoms may last from 1 week to several months. A maculopapular rash appears on the second to fifth days in more than 50% of cases. The patient exhibits erythema of the face and neck, which evolves to a macular or maculopapular exanthem of the trunk, limbs, face, palms, and soles. Pruritis is common and petechiae have been seen in some patients. Laboratory tests reveal mild leukopenia and relative lymphocytosis. Joint pain is most severe in adults, whereas children occasionally present with seizures or convulsions.

Specimens for diagnostic testing: blood (not frozen), serum

Patient isolation precautions: prevent access by mosquitoes

Suggested assays for virus detection: detection of viral RNA by RT-PCR, virus isolation in cell cultures

Serodiagnosis: enzyme-linked immunosorbent assays for IgM and IgG antibodies, neutralization tests for confirmation

Biosafety level required for working with chikungunya virus: BSL-3

Additional reading

Anon. Chikungunya fever among US Peace Corps volunteers – Republic of the Philippines. MMWR Morb Mort Wkly Rep 1986; 35:573–4.

Brighton SW, Prozesky OW, de la Harpe AL. Chikungunya virus infection. A retrospective study of 107 cases. S Afr Med J 1983;63:313–5.

Gear JH. Hemorrhagic fevers, with special reference to recent outbreaks in southern Africa. Rev Infect Dis 1979;1:571–91.

Griffin DE. Alphaviruses. In: Knipe DM, Howley PM, editors. Fields virology. Vol 1. 4th ed. Philadelphia: Lippincott Williams & Wilkins; 2001. p. 917–62.

Pile JC, Henchal EA, Christopher GW, et al. Chikungunya in a North American traveler. J Travel Med 1999;6:137–9.

Powers AM, Brault AC, Tesh RB, Weaver SC. Re-emergence of Chikungunya and O'nyong-nyong viruses: evidence for distinct geographical lineages and distant evolutionary relationships. J Gen Virol 2000;81(Pt 2):471–9.

Schlesinger S, Schlesinger MJ. Togaviridae: the viruses and their replication. In: Knipe DM, Howley PM, editors. Fields virology. Vol 1. 4th ed. Philadelphia: Lippincott Williams & Wilkins; 2001. p. 895–916.

Thaikruea L, Charearnsook O, Reanphumkarnkit S, et al. Chikungunya in Thailand: a re-emerging disease? Southeast Asian J Trop Med Public Health 1997;28:359–64.

http://www.harvardvanguard.org/kbase/nord/nord145.htm (accessed September 21, 2002).

Colorado tick fever (CTF)
(American mountain fever, Mountain fever, Mountain tick fever)

Agent: Colorado tick fever virus, family Reoviridae, genus *Coltivirus* (RNA)

Reservoir: ground squirrel, chipmunk, tick, mouse, rabbit, hare, porcupine, woodchuck

Vector: tick (*Dermacentor andersoni*)

Vehicle: none

Incubation period: 4 d–5 d (range 1 d–14 d)

Clinical hints:

- biphasic illness
- eye pain
- headache
- history of tick bite
- leukopenia
- myalgia
- pharyngitis
- photophobia
- vomiting

Typical therapy: symptomatic

Disease distribution: Canada, United States

Notes

Most cases of Colorado tick fever occur between May and July in Colorado, Idaho, Nevada, Montana, Utah, Oregon, Washington, Wyoming, eastern California, Arizona, New Mexico, and South Dakota; above 1,200 m elevation. Cases have also been reported from Alberta and British Columbia in Canada.

Only 50% of patients recall a bite from the tick vector. On rare occasions, infection has followed blood transfusion.

The principal hosts are the least chipmunk (*Tamias minimus*) and golden-mantled ground squirrel (*Citellus lateralis*).

Clinical presentation: A biphasic (50% of cases), or even triphasic (relapsing), illness may occur. Clinical features consist of maculopapular rash and fever with myalgia, headache, leukopenia, and atypical lymphocytosis. Thrombocytopenia with hemorrhagic phenomena, pharyngitis, hepatitis, myocarditis, encephalitis, orchitis, and pneumonia have been seen in some cases. The illness usually resolves in 7 to 10 days.

Specimens for diagnostic testing: whole blood (iced but unfrozen), serum

Patient isolation precautions: none

Suggested assays for virus detection: virus isolation in cell cultures or in suckling mice, detection of viral RNA by RT-PCR

Serodiagnosis: enzyme-linked immunosorbent assays for IgM and IgG antibodies, neutralization tests for confirmation

Biosafety level required for working with CTF virus: BSL-2

Additional reading

Calisher CH. Medically important arboviruses of the United States and Canada. Clin Microbiol Rev 1994;7:89–116.

Goodpasture HC, Poland JD, Francy DB, et al. Colorado tick fever: clinical, epidemiologic, and laboratory aspects of 228 cases in Colorado in 1973–1974. Ann Intern Med 1978;88:303–10.

Kettyls GD, Verrall VM, Wilton LD, et al. Arbovirus infections in man in British Columbia. Can Med Assoc J 1972;106:1175–9.

Nibert ML, Schiff LA. Reoviridae: the viruses and their replication. In: Knipe DM, Howley PM, editors. Fields virology. Vol 2. 4th ed. Philadelphia: Lippincott Williams & Wilkins; 2001. p. 1679–728.

Roy P. Orbiviruses. In: Knipe DM, Howley PM, editors. Fields virology. Vol 2. 4th ed. Philadelphia: Lippincott Williams & Wilkins; 2001. p. 1835–69.

Spruance SL, Bailey A. Colorado tick fever. A review of 115 laboratory confirmed cases. Arch Intern Med 1973;131:288–93.

Tsai TF. Arboviral infections in the United States. Infect Dis Clin North Am 1991;5:73–102.

http://www.emedicine.com/emerg/topic586.htm (accessed September 21, 2002).

Cowpox disease
(Vaccinia)

Agent: cowpox virus, family Poxviridae, genus *Orthopoxvirus* (DNA)

Reservoir: cattle, cat

Vector: none

Vehicle: cow or cat contact

Incubation period: 2 d–4 d

Clinical hints:

contact with infected animals, or smallpox vaccination
painful regional lymphadenopathy
usually on the hand
vesicles or pustules

Typical therapy: none

Disease distribution:

Germany	Russia (former Soviet Union)
India	United Kingdom
Netherlands	United States
Norway	

Notes

A variety of viruses are associated with pox-like lesions in animals: sheeppox, fowlpox, goatpox, mousepox, etc. The literature contains anecdotal, albeit unconfirmed, instances of **camelpox** among animal handlers.

Cowpox is reported primarily in Europe.

Although humans acquire infection from cows or cats, including domestic and rural animals, a rodent reservoir appears to exist in nature.

Seropositivity is found among bank voles (*Clethrionomys glareolus*) and wood mice (*Apodemus sylvaticus*).

Reservoir hosts include susliks and gerbils in the former Soviet Union, and bank voles and wood mice in the United Kingdom.

A similar illness, **buffalopox**, is encountered in India; and an emergent virus, tentatively named **Cantagalo** virus, has been described among humans and cattle in Brazil.

Clinical presentation: The infection is characterized by single or multiple vesicles of the hands or face, which evolve to pustules that may persist for 2 or more months. The surrounding tissues are swollen and painful, and tender regional adenopathy is present. Previous smallpox vaccination may attenuate the infection. Disseminated infection may occur in immune-compromised patients or individuals with eczema. Rare cases of encephalitis have been reported.

Specimens for diagnostic testing: skin exudate or biopsy

Patient isolation precautions: prevent direct contact with lesions

Suggested assays for virus detection: virus isolation in cell cultures, detection of viral nucleic acid by RT-PCR

Serodiagnosis: enzyme-linked immunosorbent assays for IgM and IgG antibodies, neutralization tests for confirmation

Biosafety level required for working with this virus: BSL-3

Additional reading

Damaso CR, Esposito JJ, Condit RC, Moussatche N. An emergent poxvirus from humans and cattle in Rio de Janeiro State: Cantagalo virus may derive from Brazilian smallpox vaccine. Virology 2000;277:439–49.

Esposito JJ, Fenner F. Poxviruses. In: Knipe DM, Howley PM, editors. Fields virology. Vol 2. 4th ed. Philadelphia: Lippincott Williams & Wilkins; 2001. p. 2885–921.

Hazel SM, Bennett M, Chantrey J, et al. A longitudinal study of an endemic disease in its wildlife reservoir: cowpox and wild rodents. Epidemiol Infect 2000;124:551–562.

Hunt E. Infectious skin diseases of cattle. Vet Clin North Am Large Anim Pract 1984;6:155–74.

Meyer H, Schay C, Mahnel H, Pfeffer M. Characterization of orthopoxviruses isolated from man and animals in Germany. Arch Virol 1999;144:491–501.

Moss B. Poxviridae: the viruses and their replication. In: Knipe DM, Howley PM, editors. Fields virology. Vol 2. 4th ed. Philadelphia: Lippincott Williams & Wilkins; 2001. p. 2849–83.

Stewart KJ, Telfer S, Bown KJ, White MI. Cowpox infection: not yet consigned to history. Br J Plast Surg 2000;53:348–50.

Crimean-Congo hemorrhagic fever (CCHF)
(Acute infectious capillary toxinosis, Xinjiang hemorrhagic fever)

Agent: Crimean-Congo hemorrhagic fever virus, family Bunyaviridae, genus *Nairovirus* (RNA), human infection by related agents (Nairobi sheep disease virus and Dugbe viruses) has been rarely reported

Reservoir: hare, bird, tick, cattle, sheep, goat

Vector: tick (*Hyalomma* spp: more than 30 potential vectors in this genus)

Vehicle: infected secretions from patient or livestock

Incubation period: 1 d–6 d (range 2 d–12 d)

Clinical hints:

abdominal pain	petechiae
chills	pharyngitis
conjunctivitis	photophobia
headache	thrombocytopenia
leukopenia	tick bite
myalgia	

Typical therapy: isolation; supportive; suggest Ribavirin 1.0 g PO qid × 4 d, then 0.5 g PO qid × 6 d

Disease distribution:

Afghanistan	China
Albania	Democratic Republic of Congo
Benin	
Bulgaria	Egypt
Burkina Faso	Ethiopia
Central African Republic	Greece

Hungary	Pakistan
India	Russia (former Soviet Union)
Iran	Saudi Arabia
Iraq	Senegal
Kenya	South Africa
Kuwait	Sudan
Madagascar	Tanzania
Mauritania	Uganda
Namibia	United Arab Emirates
Niger	Yugoslavia (former)
Nigeria	Zimbabwe
Oman	

Considered a potential bioterrorism weapon.

Notes

Crimean hemorrhagic fever was first described in the Crimea in 1944, and later equated with an illness that occurred in the Congo in 1956. Widely scattered cases were subsequently confirmed in Europe and Asia, most commonly among adult males engaged in the livestock industry. Evidence for the presence of the virus has been found among ticks in Africa, Asia, the Middle East, and Eastern Europe.

The virus is transmitted to humans through the bites of ixodid ticks (*Hyalomma* spp), or through contact with infected blood and tissues from livestock. Human-to-human transmission also occurs.

The related **Nairobi sheep disease** virus is found in India, Kenya, Ethiopia, Botswana, Mozambique, and Somalia.

Erve virus is a tick-borne nairovirus that has been associated with cases of encephalopathy and "thunder-headache" in Europe. The agent has been isolated from the tissues of white-toothed shrews (*Crocidura russula*), other insectivores, rodents, wild boars (*Sus scrofa*), red deer (*Cervus elaphus*), sheep, herring gulls (*Larus argentatus*), and humans in France, Germany, The Netherlands, and the Czech Republic.

Tribec is also tick-borne, and has been implicated in cases of meningoencephalitis.

Ganjam virus belongs to the Nairobi sheep group, and has been responsible for a case of nondescript illness acquired in an Indian laboratory.

Dugbe virus (vector: *Amblyomma variegatum*) has caused human disease in Nigeria and the Central African Republic. Antibody to this virus was also demonstrated in Senegal, Ethiopia, and Uganda.

All of the 32 members of the genus *Nairovirus* are transmitted by argasid or ixodid ticks, but only three have been definitely implicated as causes of human disease: CCHF, Dugbe, and Nairobi sheep disease viruses. CCHF virus is the most important human pathogen amongst them. The CCHF virus may infect a wide range of domestic and wild animals. Many bird species are resistant to infection, but ostriches are susceptible and may show a high prevalence of infection in endemic areas.

Animals become infected with CCHF virus from the bite of infected ticks. Ticks belonging to many genera are capable of becoming infected with CCHF virus, but the most efficient and common vectors for CCHF appear to be members of the genus *Hyalomma*. Transmission of the virus from infected female ticks to offspring via eggs (transovarial) and transmission from one sex to the other during mating (venereal) have been demonstrated amongst some vector species. The most important source for acquisition of the virus by ticks is believed to be infected small vertebrates on which immature *Hyalomma* ticks feed. Once infected, the tick remains infected through its developmental stages, and the mature tick may transmit the infection to large vertebrates, such as livestock.

Domestic ruminants can become viremic for about a week after becoming infected. Humans become infected with the CCHF virus through a tick bite or through direct contact with blood or other infected tissues from livestock. The majority of cases occur in those involved with the livestock industry, such as agricultural workers, slaughterhouse workers, and veterinarians. The virus has been found in cattle, goats, sheep, hares, and hedgehogs; livestock have subclinical infections.

Clinical presentation: The incubation period following tick bite is usually 1 to 3 days, with a maximum of 9 days; that following contact with infected blood or tissues is usually 5 to 6 days, with a maximum of 13 days.

Onset of illness is sudden, with fever, myalgia, vertigo, neck pain and stiffness, backache, headache, and photophobia. There may be initial nausea, vomiting, and sore throat accompanied by diarrhea and generalized abdominal pain. Later, the patient may experience sharp mood swings, and may become confused and aggressive. After 2 to 4 days, agitation is replaced by somnolence, depression, and lassitude, and the abdominal pain may localize to the right upper quadrant, with detectable hepatomegaly.

Other clinical signs at this stage include tachycardia, lymphadenopathy, and a petechial rash that progresses to ecchymoses and other bleeding diatheses. There is usually evidence of hepatitis. The severely ill may develop hepatorenal and pulmonary failure after the fifth day of illness.

Diagnosis of suspected CCHF is performed in specially equipped, high biosafety level laboratories. IgG and IgM antibodies may be detected in serum by enzyme-linked immunosorbent assay from day 6 of illness. IgM remains detectable for up to 4 months, and IgG levels decline but remain detectable for at least 5 years. Although an inactivated mouse brain-derived vaccine against CCHF has been developed and used on a small scale in Eastern Europe, there is no safe and effective vaccine widely available for human use.

Specimens for diagnostic testing: blood, CSF, tissue, serum

Patient isolation precautions: strict isolation

Suggested assays for virus detection: detection of viral RNA by RT-PCR, virus isolation in cell cultures

Serodiagnosis: enzyme-linked immunosorbent assays for IgM and IgG antibodies, neutralization tests for confirmation

Biosafety level required for working with CCHF virus: BSL-4

Additional reading

Fisher-Hoch SP, Khan JA, Rehman S, et al. Crimean-Congo haemorrhagic fever treated with oral ribavirin. Lancet 1995; 346:472–5.

Gear JH. Clinical aspects of African viral hemorrhagic fevers. Rev Infect Dis 1989;11 Suppl 4:S777–82.

Hassanein KM, el Azazy OM, Yousef HM. Detection of Crimean-Congo haemorrhagic fever virus antibodies in humans and imported livestock in Saudi Arabia. Trans R Soc Trop Med Hyg 1997;91:536–7.

Khan AS, Maupin GO, Rollin PE, et al. An outbreak of Crimean-Congo hemorrhagic fever in the United Arab Emirates, 1994–1995. Am J Trop Med Hyg 1997;57:519–25.

LeDuc JW. Epidemiology of hemorrhagic fever viruses. Rev Infect Dis 1989;11 Suppl 4:S730–5.

Nichol ST. Bunyaviruses. In: Knipe DM, Howley PM, editors. Fields Virology. Vol 2. 4th ed. Philadelphia: Lippincott Williams & Wilkins; 2001. p. 1603–33.

Schmaljohn CS, Hooper JW. Bunyaviridae: the viruses and their replication. In: Knipe DM, Howley PM, editors. Fields virology. Vol 2. 4th ed. Philadelphia: Lippincott Williams & Wilkins; 2001. p. 1581–602.

Schwarz TF, Nsanze H, Ameen AM. Clinical features of Crimean-Congo haemorrhagic fever in the United Arab Emirates. Infection 1997;25:364–7.

Scrimgeour EM, Mehta FR, Suleiman AJ. Infectious and tropical diseases in Oman: a review. Am J Trop Med Hyg 1999;61:920–5.

Swanepoel R, Shepherd AJ, Leman PA, et al. Epidemiologic and clinical features of Crimean-Congo hemorrhagic fever in southern Africa. Am J Trop Med Hyg 1987;36:120–32.

http://www.who.int/emc/diseases/ebola/index.html (accessed September 21, 2002).

http://www.emedicine.com/emerg/topic887.htm (accessed September 21, 2002).

Dengue fever/dengue hemorrhagic fever
(Bouquet fever, Break-bone fever, Dandy fever, Gandy fever, Date fever, Duengero, Giraffe fever, Polka fever)

Agent: any of four viruses, family Flaviviridae, genus *Flavivirus* (RNA)

Reservoir: humans, mosquito, possibly monkeys (in Malaysia and Africa)

Vector: mosquito (*Aedes aegypti*, *Aedes albopictus*, *Aedes polynesiensis*, *Aedes scutellaris*)

Vehicle: none

Incubation period: 5 d–8 d (range 2 d–15 d)

Clinical hints:

- arthralgia
- headache
- leukopenia
- macular rash
- myalgia
- relative bradycardia

Typical therapy: symptomatic

Disease distribution:

- Afghanistan
- American Samoa
- Angola
- Anguilla
- Antigua & Barbuda
- Argentina
- Aruba
- Australia
- Bahamas
- Bangladesh
- Barbados
- Belize
- Bhutan
- Bolivia
- Brazil
- British Virgin Islands
- Brunei
- Burkina Faso
- Cambodia
- China

- Colombia
- Comoros
- Cook Islands
- Costa Rica
- Cuba
- Djibouti
- Dominica
- Dominican Republic
- Ecuador
- Egypt
- El Salvador
- Fiji
- French Guiana
- French Polynesia
- Grenada
- Guadeloupe
- Guam
- Guatemala
- Guinea
- Guyana
- Haiti
- Honduras
- India
- Indonesia
- Iran
- Ivory Coast
- Jamaica
- Kenya
- Kiribati
- Laos
- Madagascar
- Malaysia
- Maldives
- Martinique
- Mauritius
- Mexico
- Montserrat
- Mozambique
- Myanmar (Burma)
- Nauru
- Nepal
- Netherlands Antilles
- New Caledonia
- Nicaragua
- Nigeria
- Niue
- Oman
- Pakistan
- Panama
- Papua New Guinea
- Paraguay
- Peru
- Philippines
- Puerto Rico
- Reunion
- Samoa
- Saudi Arabia
- Senegal
- Seychelles
- Singapore
- Solomon Islands
- Somalia
- Sri Lanka
- St. Kitts & Nevis

St. Lucia	Trust Territory Pacific Islands
St. Vincent & Grenadines	Turks and Caicos Islands
Sudan	Tuvalu
Suriname	United States
Taiwan	Vanuatu
Tanzania	Venezuela
Thailand	Vietnam
Tokelau	Virgin Islands, USA
Tonga	Wallis and Futuna Islands
Trinidad & Tobago	Yemen

Notes

As of 1998, 2.5 billion people are considered at risk for acquiring dengue, and two-thirds of the world's population live in areas infested with potential dengue virus vectors.

Estimated yearly number of cases of dengue fever (DF) have been recorded as follows: 10,000 to 300,000 cases for the period 1955 to 1959, 67.7 million in 1987, and 20.2 million to 32.3 million for the period 1994 to 1996.

Average numbers of annually-reported cases of DF were as follows: 908 cases during 1955 to 1959, 15,497 during 1960 to 1969, 122,174 during 1970 to 1979, 295,591 during 1980 to 1989, and 514,139 during 1990 to 1998.

In 1996, 3.1 million cases of DF and 138,000 deaths were reported. More than 1.2 million cases were officially reported in 1998.

In 1998, 15,000 fatal cases of dengue hemorrhagic fever (DHF) were estimated to have occurred, whereas there were 13,000 in 1999.

The risk for DHF is 0.2% during the first attack of dengue, but the risk increases 10-fold during reinfection by a second dengue serotype.

Dengue fever/dengue hemorrhagic fever

It is estimated that more than 100,000 cases of DHF occur each year worldwide.

During 1956 to 1980, there were 715,238 cases of DHF and 21,345 deaths reported worldwide, whereas 1,263,321 cases of DHF and 15,940 deaths occurred during 1986 to 1990.

The world's first recognized epidemic of DHF was reported in the Philippines during 1953 to 1954. The incidence of DHF is higher in Asia than in other dengue-endemic areas, with two-thirds of regional cases reported from Vietnam and Thailand. Over 100,000 deaths from dengue were estimated for Asia in 1995.

Dengue was first reported in the Caribbean–Latin American region in 1827, in the Virgin Islands, presumably imported with African slaves. During 1978 to 1980, 700,000 cases of dengue were reported in the American Region. Five countries in the Americas reported a total of 60 cases of DHF during 1968 to 1980. Twenty-four countries reported a total of 37,030 cases during 1981 to 1985, 65,998 in 1985, and 88,750 in 1986.

Yearly number of cases of DHF reported in the Americas were as follows: 60 cases prior to 1981, 10,312 in 1981, 3 in 1982, 0 in 1983, 8 in 1984, 12 in 1985, 35 in 1986, 97 in 1987, 86 in 1988, 2,682 in 1989, 3,646 in 1990, 2,309 in 1991, 1,753 in 1992, 4,189 in 1993, 4,177 in 1994, 9,129 in 1995, and 3,733 in 1996.

During 1981 to 1996, 42,246 cases of DHF (582 fatal) were reported in the Americas.

In Latin America, 284,483 cases of DF (7,715 DHF, 104 fatal) were reported during 1995. There were 250,707 cases (4,400 DHF, 47 fatalities) in 1996, including outbreaks in Brazil, Costa Rica, Dominican Republic, Haiti, Mexico, Nicaragua, Panama, Puerto Rico, and Venezuela. In 1997, the number of cases stood at 364,945 (10,300 DHF, 107 fatalities), in 1998 was 741,794 (72.2% of these in Brazil), and in 1999 was 259,565. 651,923 cases (15,504 DHF, 138 fatal) were reported in 2001.

In the Western Pacific region, 33 of 37 countries report dengue incidents. The numbers reported were 552,088 cases during 1993 to 1997, 131,728 (532 fatal) in 1996, 151,123 (787 fatal) in 1997, and 78,608 (246 fatal) during January to July 1998. An outbreak of 119 cases was reported in Hawaii during 2001 to 2002.

Aedes aegypti was eradicated from 21 countries in the Americas during 1948 to 1962; however, as of 1996, this mosquito is found in all countries in the area, except Bermuda, Canada, Chile, and Uruguay.

Aedes albopictus, a potential vector, has recently been found in Europe, surfacing in Albania in 1976 and in Italy in 1990 and in Israel in 2002. As of 1996, *Ae. albopictus* is also present in six countries in the American continent: Brazil, the Dominican Republic, El Salvador, Guatemala, Mexico, and the United States.

Aedes polynesiensis has also been implicated as a dengue vector.

The first dengue viruses recognized in Africa were isolated during 1964 to 1968, in Nigeria. Serosurveys suggest that DF is hyperendemic in certain areas of West Africa, and probably East Africa as well. Many cases are probably misdiagnosed as malaria.

Clinical presentation: For surveillance purposes, the US Centers for Disease Control and Prevention (CDC) defines DF as an "acute febrile illness characterized by frontal headache, retro-ocular pain, muscle and joint pain, and rash." The initial fever rises rapidly and lasts for 2 to 7 days. Occasionally, it may have a "saddle-back" appearance with a drop after a few days, and rebound within 24 hours. Conjunctival injection and pharyngeal inflammation may occur, as well as lymphadenopathy. Rash occurs in up to 50% of patients, either early in the illness with flushing or mottling, or between the second to the sixth day as a scarlatiniform or maculopapular rash that usually spreads centrifugally. The later rash usually lasts for 2 to 3 days. Diffuse erythema and late desquamation of the hands and feet may be confused with toxic shock syndrome. As fever drops, petechiae may be seen. For a diagnosis of DHF to be made, the presence of thrombocytopenia ($<100,000/mm^3$) and evidence of plasma leakage (hematocrit increased by at least 20%) or other objective evidence of increased capillary permeability are required. Dengue shock syndrome consists of DHF in addition to hypotension or narrow pulse pressure of less than 21 mm Hg.

Specimens for diagnostic testing: serum, tissue

Patient isolation precautions: prevent access by mosquitoes

Suggested assays for virus detection: detection of viral RNA by RT-PCR, virus isolation in mosquitoes or in mosquito cell cultures

Serodiagnosis: enzyme-linked immunosorbent assays for IgM and IgG antibodies, neutralization tests for confirmation

Biosafety level required for working with dengue viruses: BSL-2

Additional reading

Anon. Dengue/dengue haemorrhagic fever. Wkly Epidemiol Rec 2000;75:193–6.

Anon. Imported dengue — United States, 1997 and 1998. MMWR Morb Mort Wkly Rep 2000;49:248–53.

Burke DS, Monath TP. Flaviviruses. In: Knipe DM, Howley PM, editors. Fields virology. Vol 1. 4th ed. Philadelphia: Lippincott Williams & Wilkins; 2001. p. 1043–126.

Githeko AK, Lindsay SW, Confalonieri UE, Patz JA. Climate change and vector-borne diseases: a regional analysis. Bull World Health Organ 2000;78:1136–47.

Gubler DJ. Dengue and dengue hemorrhagic fever. Clin Microbiol Rev 1998;11:480–96.

Isturiz RE, Gubler DJ, Brea del Castillo J. Dengue and dengue hemorrhagic fever in Latin America and the Caribbean. Infect Dis Clin North Am 2000;14:121–40.

Jacobs M. Dengue: emergence as a global public health problem and prospects for control. Trans R Soc Trop Med Hyg 2000;94:7–8.

Lindenbach BD, Rice CM. Flaviviridae: the viruses and their replication. In: Knipe DM, Howley PM, editors. Fields virology. Vol 1. 4th ed. Philadelphia: Lippincott Williams & Wilkins; 2001. p. 991–1041.

Rigau Perez JG, Clark GG, Gubler DJ, et al. Dengue and dengue haemorrhagic fever. Lancet 1998;352:971–7.

http://www.who.int/emc/diseases/ebola/index.html (accessed September 21, 2002)

http://www.cdc.gov/ncidod/diseases/submenus/sub_dengue.htm (accessed September 21, 2002).

http://www.emedicine.com/emerg/topic124.htm (accessed September 21, 2002).

Eastern equine encephalitis (EEE)

Agent: eastern equine encephalitis virus, family Togaviridae, genus *Alphavirus* (RNA)

Reservoir: wild birds, horses, pigs

Vector: mosquito (*Aedes* spp, *Culiseta* spp)

Vehicle: direct patient contact

Incubation period: 7 d–10 d (range 5 d–15 d)

Clinical hints:

- coma
- fever
- headache
- leukocytosis
- neurological findings
- seizures
- summer illness (in temperate areas)

Typical therapy: symptomatic

Disease distribution:

- Argentina
- Belize
- Brazil
- Canada
- Colombia
- Cuba
- Dominican Republic
- Ecuador
- El Salvador
- Guatemala
- Guyana
- Honduras
- Jamaica
- Mexico
- Panama
- Peru
- Suriname
- United States (Figure 4)
- Venezuela

Considered a potential bioterrorism weapon.

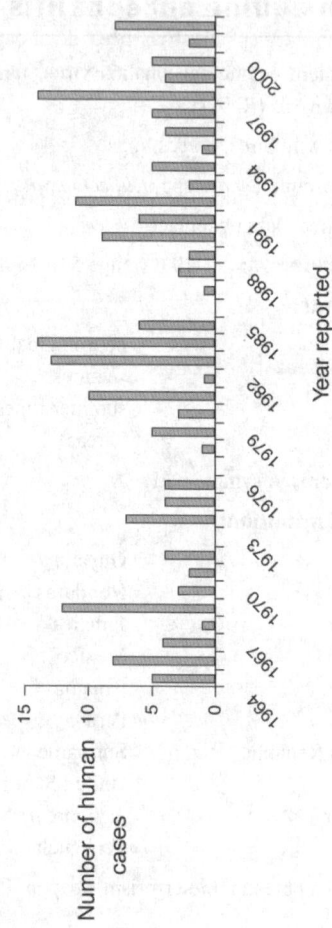

Figure 4 Eastern equine encephalitis in the United States.

Notes

Eastern equine encephalitis has been documented throughout North and Central America, the Caribbean, and as far south as Argentina.

Though relatively rare, human infection is often severe or fatal, with major neurological sequelae in 50 to 70% of cases. Asymptomatic infection is reported in approximately 95% of infected adults, and in 85% of infected children.

Most infections in North America are reported from coastal regions, during the summer months. Increasing death of local horses may herald local outbreaks.

Clinical presentation: Clinical features of eastern equine encephalitis (EEE), western equine encephalitis (WEE), and Venezuelan equine encephalitis (VEE) are similar, and will be discussed as a group. EEE and WEE virus infections begin with headache, high fever, chills, and vomiting. Vertigo, sore throat, and respiratory symptoms are common in WEE virus infection. Central nervous system involvement is heralded by confusion and somnolence, which may progress to coma. Focal or generalized seizures are most common in younger patients. Physical examination reveals nuchal rigidity, depressed or hyperactive reflexes, tremors, or spastic paralysis. The peripheral blood reveals leukocytosis, which is more prominent in EEE than in WEE. Cerebrospinal fluid protein levels are elevated. WEE tends to produce a lymphocytic pleocytosis of 50 to $500/mm^3$, whereas that from EEE is 600 to $2,000/mm^3$. Sequelae are most severe following EEE virus infection, and include mental retardation, behavioral changes, seizure disorders, and paralysis. Sequelae occur in 30% of infants recovering from WEE, and in 70% of infants recovering from EEE. Parkinsonism may occur in adults following WEE. Case-fatality rates of as high as 70% have been reported for EEE.

VEE is often characterized by a mild flu-like illness in endemic countries. Overt infection is heralded by fever, chills, myalgia, headache with or without photophobia, hyperesthesia, and vomiting. Sore throat is noted in some cases. Four percent of children and less than 1% of adults progress to overt encephalitis, a few days to a week following the prodrome. Encephalitis is characterized by nuchal rigidity, ataxia, convulsions, coma, and paralysis. Lymphopenia is common, and often associated with neutropenia and mild thrombocytopenia. Hepatic dysfunction is also common, and CSF examination reveals a few hundred lymphocytes. The case-fatality rate is less than 1%, but increases to 20% in cases of encephalitis.

Specimens for diagnostic testing: brain tissue, CSF, serum

Patient isolation precautions: none

Suggested assays for virus detection: detection of viral RNA by RT-PCR, virus isolation in cell cultures

Serodiagnosis: enzyme-linked immunosorbent assays for IgM and IgG antibodies, neutralization tests for confirmation

Biosafety level required for working with eastern equine encephalitis virus: BSL-2

Additional reading

Anon. Arboviral disease — United States, 1994. MMWR Morb Mort Wkly Rep 1995;44:641–4.

Calisher CH. Medically important arboviruses of the United States and Canada. Clin Microbiol Rev 1994;7:89–116.

Deresiewicz RL, Thaler SJ, Hsu L, Zamani AA. Clinical and neuroradiographic manifestations of eastern equine encephalitis. N Engl J Med 1997;336:1867–74.

Freier JE. Eastern equine encephalomyelitis. Lancet 1993;342: 1281–2.

Griffin DE. Alphaviruses. In: Knipe DM, Howley PM, editors. Fields virology. Vol 1. 4th ed. Philadelphia: Lippincott Williams & Wilkins; 2001. p. 917–62.

Gutierrez KM, Prober CG. Encephalitis. Identifying the specific cause is key to effective management. Postgrad Med 1998;103:123–5, 129–30, 140–3.

Letson GW, Bailey RE, Pearson J, Tsai TF. Eastern equine encephalitis (EEE): a description of the 1989 outbreak, recent epidemiologic trends, and the association of rainfall with EEE occurrence. Am J Trop Med Hyg 1993;49:677–85.

Nasci RS, Moore CG. Vector-borne disease surveillance and natural disasters. Emerg Infect Dis 1998;4:333–4.

Schlesinger S, Schlesinger MJ. Togaviridae: the viruses and their replication. In: Knipe DM, Howley PM, editors. Fields virology. Vol 1. 4th ed. Philadelphia: Lippincott Williams & Wilkins; 2001. p. 895–916.

Tsai TF. Arboviral infections in the United States. Infect Dis Clin North Am 1991;5:73–102.

http://www.cdc.gov/ncidod/dvbid/arbor/index.htm (accessed September 21, 2002).

http://www.cdc.gov/ncidod/diseases/list_mosquitoborne.htm (accessed September 21, 2002).

Ebola hemorrhagic fever

Agent: any one of a number of closely related viruses, family Filoviridae, genus *Ebolavirus* (RNA)

Reservoir: unknown

Vector: none

Vehicle: secretions, contact, contaminated needle or syringe

Incubation period: 5 d–12 d (range 2 d–21 d)

Clinical hints:

arthralgia	hepatic dysfunction
conjunctivitis	maculopapular rash
diarrhea	myalgia
fever	sore throat
hemorrhagic diatheses	vomiting

Typical therapy: symptomatic

Disease distribution:

Central African Republic	Liberia
Democratic Republic of Congo	Madagascar
Ethiopia	Nigeria
Gabon	Sudan
Guinea	Uganda
Ivory Coast	Zimbabwe
Kenya	

Considered a potential bioterrorism weapon.

Notes

Ebola was first identified in June 1976, during an outbreak in Sudan that involved 284 cases with fatality of 53%. In September 1976, a separate outbreak was reported from Zaire (Democratic Republic of the Congo) involving 318 cases, 88% of which were fatal. An additional fatal case was identified in that country in June 1977.

An outbreak of 34 cases was reported in Sudan in 1979, 64% of which were fatal. The disease was not identified again until 1994, when outbreaks occurred in Cote d'Ivoire in 12 chimpanzees and one human, and in Gabon, where 59% of the 49 cases were fatal.

In 1995, 315 cases were reported in the Democratic Republic of the Congo, of which 77% were fatal.

In 1996, two outbreaks were reported in Gabon: one of 31 cases, 68% fatalities and the other of 60 cases, 75% fatalities.

In 2000, 428 cases were reported in Uganda, of which 160 were fatal.

During 2001 to 2002, 100 cases were reported in Gabon and in neighboring areas of Congo, of which 74 were fatal.

In 1989, a related virus (Reston strain) was identified in monkeys (cynomolgus macaques) imported from the Philippines to the United States. At least four human contacts seroconverted without clinical illness. Two imported monkeys from the Philippines died of Ebola in Texas, in 1996.

Four ebolaviruses have been described: Ivory Coast, Reston, Sudan, and Zaire.

Clinical presentation: The symptoms and signs of infection with Ebola and Marburg viruses (family Filoviridae, genus *Marburgvirus*) are similar. Following an incubation period of 4 to 16 days, onset is sudden, marked by anorexia, fever, chills, headache, and myalgia. Later, the patient develops nausea, vomiting, sore throat, abdominal pain, and diarrhea. Patients are dehydrated, apathetic, and disoriented, and exhibit pharyngeal and conjunctival injection. Most develop severe hemorrhagic manifestations between days 5 and 7. Bleeding is often from multiple sites, most commonly from the gastrointestinal tract, lungs, and gingiva. Hemorrhage and oropharyngeal lesions carry a particularly poor prognosis. Death occurs between days 7 and 16. Case-fatality rates of 50 to 90% are reported.

Specimens for diagnostic testing: blood, serum, liver, spleen

Patient isolation precautions: strict isolation

Suggested assays for virus detection: detection of viral RNA by RT-PCR, virus isolation not recommended

Serodiagnosis: enzyme-linked immunosorbent assays and immunofluorescence assays for IgM and IgG antibodies

Biosafety level required for working with Ebola virus: BSL-4

Additional reading

Anon. Ebola: the virus and the disease. Wkly Epidemiol Rec 1999;74:89.

Colebunders R, Borchert M. Ebola haemorrhagic fever — a review. J Infect 2000;40:16–20.

DeMarcus TA, Tipple MA, Ostrowski SR. US policy for disease control among imported nonhuman primates. J Infect Dis 1999;179 Suppl 1:S281–2.

Freedman DO, Woodall J. Emerging infectious diseases and risk to the traveler. Med Clin North Am 1999;83:865–83.

Khan AS, Tshioko FK, Heymann DL, et al. The reemergence of Ebola hemorrhagic fever, Democratic Republic of the Congo, 1995. Commission de Lutte contre les Epidemies a Kikwit. J Infect Dis 1999;179 Suppl 1:S76–86.

Miranda ME, Ksiazek TG, Retuya TJ, et al. Epidemiology of Ebola (subtype Reston) virus in the Philippines, 1996. J Infect Dis 1999;179 Suppl 1:S115–9.

Ndambi R, Akamituna P, Bonnet MJ, et al. Epidemiologic and clinical aspects of the Ebola virus epidemic in Mosango, Democratic Republic of the Congo, 1995. J Infect Dis 1999;179 Suppl 1: S8–10.

Sanchez A, Khan AS, Zaki SR, et al. Filoviridae: Marburg and Ebola viruses. In: Knipe DM, Howley PM, editors. Fields virology. Vol 1. 4th ed. Philadelphia: Lippincott Williams & Wilkins; 2001. p. 1279–304.

Sanchez A, Ksiazek TG, Rollin PE, et al. Reemergence of Ebola virus in Africa [editorial]. Emerg Infect Dis 1995;1:96–7.

Tomori O, Bertolli J, Rollin PE, et al. Serologic survey among hospital and health center workers during the Ebola hemorrhagic fever outbreak in Kikwit, Democratic Republic of the Congo, 1995. J Infect Dis 1999;179 Suppl 1:S98–101.

http://www.who.int/emc/diseases/ebola/index.html (accessed September 21, 2002).

http://www.cdc.gov/ncidod/diseases/virlfvr/virlfvr.htm (accessed September 21, 2002).

http://www.emedicine.com/emerg/topic887.htm (accessed September 21, 2002).

Group C viral fevers

Agent: any of a number of viruses of the family Bunyaviridae, genus *Orthobunyavirus* (RNA), Group C serogroup

Reservoir: rodent, marsupial, possibly bat

Vector: mosquito (*Culex, Aedes, Limatus, Wyeomyia, Coquillettidia, Mansonia,* and *Psorophora* spp)

Vehicle: none

Incubation period: 3 d–12 d

Clinical hints:

conjunctivitis	myalgia
exposure to forested areas	photophobia
fever	self-limited illness

Typical therapy: symptomatic

Disease distribution:

Brazil	Panama
French Guiana	Peru
Guyana	Suriname
Mexico	Trinidad & Tobago

Notes

Group C viral infections are limited to Latin America and the Caribbean. The diseases and their vectors are as follows:

Apeu: *Aedes arborealis, Aedes septemstriatus, Aedes serratus, Culex ocossa*

Caraparu: *Culex caudelli, Culex portesi, Culex spissipes, Culex vomerifer, Limatus durhamii, Wyeomyia* spp

Catu: *Anopheles nimbus, Coquillettidia venezuelensis, Culex mojuensis, Culex declarator, Culex vomerifer*

Guama: *Aedes sexlineatus, Coquillettidia venezuelensis, Cx. mojuensis, Culex epanatasis, Cx. portesi, Cx. spissipes, Culex taeniopus, Cx. vomerifer, Limatus durhamii, Wyeomyia* spp

Itaqui: *Cx. portesi, Cx. vomerifer*

Madrid: *Cx. vomerifer*

Marituba: *Cx. ocossa, Cx. portesi*

Murutucu: *Coquillettidia venezuelensis, Cx. ocossa, Cx. portesi, Sabethini* spp

Oriboca: *Aedes taeniorhynchus, Cx. portesi, Psorophora ferox, Mansonia* spp

Ossa: *Cx. taeniopus, Cx. vomerifer*

Restan: *Cx. portesi*

Clinical presentation: Abrupt onset of fever, lasting 2 to 5 days, is associated with severe headache, vertigo, nausea, myalgia, and arthralgia; a rash may occur.

Specimens for diagnostic testing: serum

Patient isolation precautions: prevent access by mosquitoes

Suggested assays for virus detection: virus isolation in cell cultures

Serodiagnosis: enzyme-linked immunosorbent assays for IgM and IgG antibodies, neutralization tests for confirmation

Biosafety level required for working with these viruses: BSL-2

Additional reading

Calisher CH, Coimbra TL, de S Lopez O, et al. Identification of new Guama and Group C serogroup bunyaviruses and an ungrouped virus from Southern Brazil. Am J Trop Med Hyg 1983;32:424–31.

De Haas RA, Arron-Leeuwin AE. Arboviruses isolated from mosquitoes and man in Surinam. Trop Geogr Med 1975;27:409–12.

De Haas RA, Timers WC. Infection rate of arboviruses in Dutch recruits returning from Surinam. Trop Geogr Med 1976;28: 137–40.

Iversson LB, Travassos da Rosa AP, Coimbra TL, et al. Human disease in Ribeira Valley, Brazil caused by Carapuru, a group C arbovirus — report of a case. Rev Inst Med Trop Sao Paulo 1987;29:112–7.

Nichol ST. Bunyaviruses. In: Knipe DM, Howley PM, editors. Fields virology. Vol 2. 4th ed. Philadelphia: Lippincott Williams & Wilkins; 2001. p. 1603–33.

Price JL. Serological evidence of infection of Tacaribe virus and arboviruses in Trinidadian bats. Am J Trop Med Hyg 1978;27: 162–7.

Scherer WF, Madalengoitia J, Flores W, Acosta M. The first isolations of eastern encephalitis, group C, and Guama group arboviruses from the Peruvian Amazon region of western South America. Bull Pan Am Health Organ 1975;9:19–26.

Schmaljohn CS, Hooper JW. Bunyaviridae: the viruses and their replication. In: Knipe DM, Howley PM, editors. Fields virology. Vol 2. 4th ed. Philadelphia: Lippincott Williams & Wilkins; 2001. p. 1581–602.

Tikasingh ES, Ardoin P, Williams MC. First isolation of Catu virus from a human in Trinidad. Trop Geogr Med 1974;26: 414–6.

Walder R, Suarez OM, Calisher CH. Arbovirus studies in southwestern Venezuela during 1973–1981. II. Isolations and further studies of Venezuelan and eastern equine encephalitis, Una, Itaqui, and Moju viruses. Am J Trop Med Hyg 1984;33:483–91.

Hantavirus infections (New World)
(Hantavirus pulmonary syndrome)

Agent: any of a number of viruses of the family Bunyaviridae, genus *Hantavirus* (RNA), including Sin Nombre, Andes, Bayou, Black Creek Canal, New York-1, and others

Reservoir: rodents: deer mouse (*Peromyscus maniculatus*-Sin Nombre), piñon mouse (*Peromyscus truei*-Sin Nombre), brush mouse (*Peromyscus boylii*-Limeston Canyon), hispid cotton rat (*Sigmodon hispidus*-Black Creek Canal), rice rat (*Oryzomys palustris*-Bayou), others (see below)

Vector: none

Vehicle: aerosols of secretions, bite or direct contact (rare), human-to-human (rare)

Incubation period: 9 d–35 d

Clinical hints:

bilateral interstitial infiltrates	fever
exposure (agriculture, hiking, rodents)	hypoxia
	myalgia
	rapidly progressive illness

Typical therapy: symptomatic

Disease distribution:

- Argentina
- Bolivia
- Brazil
- Canada
- Chile
- Colombia
- Mexico
- Panama
- Paraguay
- Peru
- United States (Figure 5)
- Uruguay
- Venezuela

Considered a potential bioterrorism weapon.

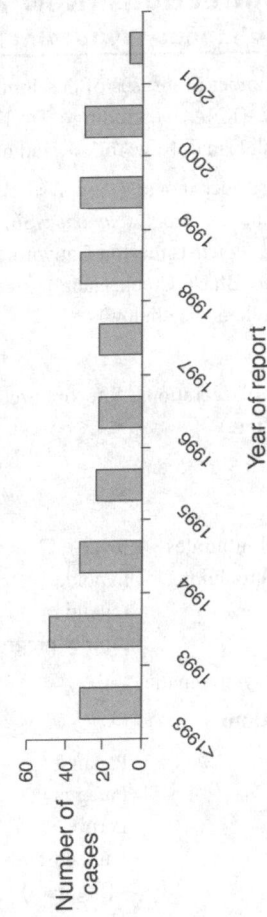

Figure 5 Hantavirus pulmonary syndrome in the United States.

Notes

After first recognition in 1993, the majority of hantavirus pulmonary syndrome (HPS) cases have been identified in the United States. As of February 2000, 316 cases were identified in North America and more than 550 cases in Central and South America.

To date, the male:female ratio for reported cases is 1.47:1, with an age range of 10 to 75 years (mean 38 years). Caucasians have accounted for 77.2% of cases, Native Americans for 19.9%, Blacks for 1.8%, and Asians for 1.1%.

Sin Nombre virus is transmitted by the deer mouse (*P. maniculatus*) in the United States, mainly in the southwest. The reservoir is found in areas stretching from the Alaska panhandle and Canada, across northern Mexico, most of the continental United States, to southernmost Baja California and north-central Oaxaca, Mexico. The mouse itself shows little evidence of disease. The virus has also been found in or on *P. truei*. **Convict Creek** virus, essentially identical to Sin Nombre virus, has been identified in California, and was implicated in a fatal HPS case there.

New York-1 virus is transmitted by the white-footed mouse (*Peromyscus leucopus*), found in regions of Central and Eastern America, and in southern Ontario, southern Alberta, Quebec, and Nova Scotia in Canada, as well as in northern Durango and along the Caribbean coast of Mexico to the Isthmus of Tehuantepec and Yucatan Peninsula.

Black Creek Canal virus is transmitted by the cotton rat (*S. hispidus*), found in US areas ranging from eastern Colorado and southern Nebraska to central Virginia, and south to southeastern Arizona and peninsular Florida. It is also found from central to eastern Mexico, in areas ranging through Central America and central Panama to northern Colombia and northern Venezuela.

Bayou virus is transmitted by the rice rat (*O. palustris*), found in Louisiana and eastern Texas to Kansas, New Jersey, and Florida.

Monongahela virus, a variant of Sin Nombre virus, is found in the eastern United States and Canada, and is carried by the white-footed mouse (*P. leucopus*) and by *P. maniculatus nubiterrae*.

Andes virus is transmitted by the long-tailed pygmy rice rat (*Oligoryzomys longicaudatus*), found in the north-central to southern Andes, Chile, Argentina, and possibly Uruguay.

Laguna Negra virus has caused human disease in Paraguay and Chile, and is transmitted by the vesper mouse (*Calomys laucha*). This rodent is found in northern Argentina and Uruguay, southeastern Bolivia, western Paraguay, west-central Brazil, and Chile.

Oran (reservoir: *Ol. longicaudatus*), **Lechiguanas** (reservoir: *Oligoryzomys flavescens*), and the unnamed HU-39694 viruses are found in Argentina.

Choclo (reservoir: *Oligoryzomys fulvescens*) virus has been implicated in HPS cases in Panama.

Juquitiba virus has been implicated in human infections in Brazil. **Bermejo** virus (reservoir *Oligoryzomys* spp) has been associated with human infections in Bolivia. **Rio Mamore** virus (reservoir *Neacomys spinosus*) has been associated with human infections in Bolivia. **Cano Delgadito** virus (clinical significance unknown) has been found in rodents in central Venezuela. **Calabazo virus** (clinical significance unknown) has been identified in *Zygodontomys brevicauda* in Panama.

Clinical presentation: The clinical case definition consists of fever of greater than 38.3°C as well as bilateral diffuse pulmonary infiltrates with respiratory compromise requiring supplemental oxygen within 72 hours of hospitalization. Fatal cases are defined as unexplained fatal respiratory illness with noncardiogenic pulmonary edema. Recently, cases of prodromic infection without severe pulmonary disease have been reported. The typical illness is characterized by fever, chills, headache and, occasionally, gastrointestinal symptoms. Five days after onset, patients develop dyspnea, with rapid progression to pulmonary edema within as few as 24 hours. The case-fatality rate is 45 to 50%.

Specimens for diagnostic testing: serum

Patient isolation precautions: limit contact with others (for lack of contradicting information)

Suggested assays for virus detection: detection of viral RNA by RT-PCR

Serodiagnosis: enzyme-linked immunosorbent assays for IgM and IgG antibodies

Biosafety level required for working with these viruses: BSL-3

Additional reading

Anon. Hantavirus in the Americas. Wkly Epidemiol Rec 1999;74:173.

Anon. Update: hantavirus pulmonary syndrome — United States, 1999. MMWR Morb Mort Wkly Rep 1999;48:521–5.

Boone JD, McGwire KC, Otteson EW, et al. Remote sensing and geographic information systems: charting Sin Nombre virus infections in deer mice. Emerg Infect Dis 2000;6:248–58.

Enria DA, Pinheiro F. Rodent-borne emerging viral zoonoses. Hemorrhagic fevers and hantavirus infections in South America. Infect Dis Clin North Am 2000;14:167–84.

Hjelle B, Glass GE. Outbreak of hantavirus infection in the Four Corners region of the United States in the wake of the

1997–1998 El Nino-southern oscillation. J Infect Dis 2000; 181:1569–73.

Mills JN, Ksiazek TG, Peters CJ, Childs JE. Long-term studies of hantavirus reservoir populations in the Southwestern United States: a synthesis. Emerg Infect Dis 1999;5:41–8.

Nichol ST. Bunyaviruses. In: Knipe DM, Howley PM, editors. Fields virology. Vol 2. 4th ed. Philadelphia: Lippincott Williams & Wilkins; 2001. p. 1603–33.

Padula PJ, Colavecchia SB, Martinez VP, et al. Genetic diversity, distribution, and serological features of hantavirus infection in five countries in South America. J Clin Microbiol 2000;38:3029–35.

Schmaljohn CS, Hooper JW. Bunyaviridae: the viruses and their replication. In: Knipe DM, Howley PM, editors. Fields virology. Vol 2. 4th ed. Philadelphia: Lippincott Williams & Wilkins; 2001. p. 1581–602.

Shope RE. A midcourse assessment of hantavirus pulmonary syndrome. Emerg Infect Dis 1999;5:172–4.

http://www.cdc.gov/ncidod/diseases/hanta/hantvrus.htm (accessed September 21, 2002).

http://www.emedicine.com/emerg/topic861.htm (accessed September 21, 2002).

Hantavirus infections (Old World)
(Acute epidemic hemorrhagic fever, Bosnian hemorrhagic fever, Churilov disease, Dobrava-Belgrade virus infection, Endemic benign nephropathy, Epidemic hemorrhagic fever, Far eastern hemorrhagic fever, Hemorrhagic nephrosonephritis, Hemorrhagic fever with renal syndrome, Infectious hemorrhagic fever, Khabarovsk disease, Korean hemorrhagic fever, Muroid virus nephropathy, Nephropathia epidemica, Rodent-borne viral nephropathy, Scandinavian epidemic nephropathy, Songo fever, Topografov disease, Viral hemorrhagic fever)

Agent: any of a number of viruses of the family Bunyaviridae, genus *Hantavirus* (RNA); includes Hantaan, Puumala, Dobrava, and Seoul viruses

Reservoir: field mouse (*Apodemus agrarius*-Hantaan), vole (*Clethrionomys glareolus*-Puumala), rat (*Rattus norvegicus*-Seoul), possibly bat, possibly bird

Vector: none

Vehicle: animal secretions

Incubation period: 12 d–21 d (range 4 d–42 d)

Clinical hints:

azotemia	hemorrhage
backache	local rodent infestation
conjunctivitis	myalgia
diarrhea	proteinuria
headache	thrombocytopenia
	vomiting

Typical therapy: symptomatic

Disease distribution:

Afghanistan
Albania
Andorra
Austria
Bangladesh
Belgium
Benin
Bhutan
Bulgaria
Burkina Faso
Cambodia
Central African Republic
China
Czechoslovakia (former)
Democratic Republic of Congo
Denmark
Egypt
Estonia
Fiji
Finland
France
Gabon
Germany
Greece
Hong Kong
Hungary
India
Indonesia
Iran
Italy
Japan
Kenya
Korea
Laos
Macao
Madagascar
Malaysia
Malta
Mauritania
Mongolia
Myanmar
Nepal
Netherlands
Nigeria
Norway
Pakistan
Papua New Guinea
Philippines
Poland
Portugal
Romania
Russia (former Soviet Union)
Rwanda
San Marino
Senegal
Singapore
South Africa

Spain	Thailand
Sri Lanka	Turkey
Sudan	Uganda
Sweden	United Kingdom
Switzerland	Vietnam
Taiwan	Yugoslavia (former)

Considered a potential bioterrorism weapon.

Notes

Infections with Old World hantaviruses are most common among agrarian and military populations. Each year, 150,000 are hospitalized, and 4,500 to 22,550 die of these infections, with more than 50% of these cases occurring in China. Approximately 200,000 cases are estimated to occur each year in Eurasia.

Hantaan virus causes hemorrhagic fever with renal syndrome (HFRS = epidemic hemorrhagic fever, Korean hemorrhagic fever). The reservoir, the striped field mouse (*A. agrarius*), is found in areas from the south of Central Europe to Thrace, the Caucasus and Tien Shan Mountains, the Amur River to East Xizang, and East Hunnan, West Sichuan, Fujian, and Taiwan.

Dobrava-Belgrade virus causes severe HFRS. The reservoir, the yellow-necked mouse (*Apodemus flavicollis*), is found in areas ranging from England and Wales, through Northwest Spain, France, southern Scandinavia, European Russia to the Urals, southern Italy, the Balkans, Syria, Lebanon, and Israel. The case-fatality rate for Dobrava virus infection is about 15%.

Seoul virus causes less severe HFRS. The reservoir rat (*R. norvegicus*) is found worldwide.

Puumala virus causes nephropathia epidemica. The reservoir, the bank vole (*C. glariolus*), is found in the West Palearctic, from France and Scandinavia to Lake Baikal, south to northern

Spain, northern Italy, the Balkans, western Turkey, northern Kazakhstan, the Altai and Sayan Mountains, Great Britain and southwestern Ireland. The house mouse (*Mus musculus*) has been implicated in Serbia, *Clethrionomys rutilis* in western Russia, and the muskrat (*Ondatra zibethicus*) in Germany. The case-fatality rate for Puumala virus infection is about 0.1%.

As of 2000, there were no proven cases of Hantaan or Seoul virus infections from Europe or from western Russia (west of the Urals); all cases reported in these areas have been caused by Dobrava virus. The Dobrava or Puumala virus has been confirmed in the former Yugoslavia, Albania, Greece, Germany, Estonia, and Russia. In contrast to the Balkan region, where Dobrova virus seems to be carried mainly by *A. flavicollis*, the virus has only been found in *A. agrarius* in Estonia and Russia. Saaremaa virus, similar to Dobrova virus, has been associated with human disease in Estonia.

Notably, two outbreaks of HFRS in the Ryazan and Tula regions in Russia that were previously reported as being caused by Seoul virus, were later proven to be caused solely by Dobrava virus.

Simultaneous HFRS epidemics in Bashkortostan (Bashkiria), Samara, and Tatarstan appear to have been related. Recent increases in the number of human cases have been ascribed to a construction boom in forests during the last decade.

Clinical presentation: The course of severe HFRS involves five overlapping stages: febrile, hypotensive, oliguric, diuretic, and convalescent; however, it is not uncommon for one or more of these stages to be inapparent or absent. The onset of the disease is sudden, with intense headache, backache, fever, and chills. Hemorrhage is manifested during the febrile phase as a flushing of the face, or injection of the conjunctiva and mucous membranes. A petechial rash may appear on the palate and axillary skin folds. Extreme albuminuria, typically appearing on the fourth day, is characteristic of severe HFRS. As the febrile stage ends, hypotension may develop and last for hours to days, accompanied by nausea and vomiting. One-third of deaths occur during this phase, related to vascular leakage and shock. Approximately 50% of deaths occur during the subsequent (oliguric) phase. Patients who survive and progress to the diuretic phase show improved renal function, but may still die of shock or pulmonary complications. The final (convalescent) phase can last weeks to months.

Case-fatality rates range from less than 0.1%, for HFRS caused by Puumala virus, to approximately 5 to 10%, for HFRS caused by Hantaan virus.

Specimens for diagnostic testing: serum

Patient isolation precautions: none

Suggested assays for virus detection: detection of viral RNA by RT-PCR

Serodiagnosis: enzyme-linked immunosorbent assays for IgM and IgG antibodies

Biosafety level required for working with these viruses: BSL-3

Additional reading

Anon. Tick-borne encephalitis and haemorrhagic fever with renal syndrome in Europe. Report on a WHO meeting. EURO Rep Stud 1986:1–79.

Brummer-Korvenkontio M, Vapalahti O, Henttonen H, et al. Epidemiological study of nephropathia epidemica in Finland 1989–96. Scand J Infect Dis 1999;31:427–35.

Clement J, Heyman P, McKenna P, et al. The hantaviruses of Europe: from the bedside to the bench. Emerg Infect Dis 1997;3:205–11.

Mustonen J, Vapalahti O, Henttonen H, et al. Epidemiology of hantavirus infections in Europe [editorial]. Nephrol Dial Transplant1998;13:2729–31.

Nichol ST. Bunyaviruses. In: Knipe DM, Howley PM, editors. Fields virology. Vol 2. 4th ed. Philadelphia: Lippincott Williams & Wilkins; 2001. p. 1603–33.

Schmaljohn CS, Hooper JW. Bunyaviridae: the viruses and their replication. In: Knipe DM, Howley PM, editors. Fields virology. Vol 2. 4th ed. Philadelphia: Lippincott Williams & Wilkins; 2001. p. 1581–602.

Settergren B. Clinical aspects of nephropathia epidemica (Puumala virus infection) in Europe: a review. Scand J Infect Dis 2000;32:125–32.

Sibold C, Meisel H, Lundkvist A, et al. Short report: simultaneous occurrence of Dobrava, Puumala, and Tula hantaviruses in Slovakia. Am J Trop Med Hyg 1999;61:409–11.

http://www.emedicine.com/emerg/topic887.htm (accessed September 21, 2002).

Hendra disease
(Bat paramyxovirus, Equine morbillivirus)

Agent: Hendra virus, family Paramyxoviridae, genus not yet assigned (RNA)

Reservoir: horse, fruit bats (*Pteropus* spp)

Vector: unknown

Vehicle: unknown, possibly urine and secretions

Incubation period: unknown

Clinical hints:

flu-like illness
follows close contact with horses
giant cell pneumonia
headache
respiratory distress
vertigo

Typical therapy: possibly Ribavirin (investigational)

Disease distribution: Australia

Notes

Hendra is a suburb of Brisbane, Queensland, Australia. A single outbreak of Hendra virus infection was described there in 1994, involving 21 horses with 14 fatalities, and two human handlers with one fatality.

Additional fatal infections were reported in 1995 in two horses and in a farmer from Mackay, North Queensland. Fatal infection in a horse was reported from Cairns in 1999.

The presumed reservoirs of Hendra virus are fruit bats (*Pteropus* spp); however, cats and guinea pigs may also be infected. A 20% seroprevalence rate has been found among pteropid bats in Queensland. In one study, none of 128 persons who care for local bats was found to be seropositive.

A second paramyxovirus, **Menangle** virus, is rarely acquired by humans in Australia. The virus causes stillbirth and deformities in piglets, and a flu-like illness with rash in humans, and it appears to have a reservoir in fruit bats.

Clinical presentation: To date only three cases of human infection by Hendra virus have been reported, thus the clinical features are largely unknown. Reported findings include headache, cough, veritgo, and respiratory distress. A diffuse infiltrate may be seen on chest x-ray, and giant cell pneumonia has been found in lung tissue.

Specimens for diagnostic testing: serum

Patient isolation precautions: limit access to others

Suggested assays for virus detection: detection of viral RNA by RT-PCR

Serodiagnosis: enzyme-linked immunosorbent assays for IgM and IgG antibodies, neutralization tests for confirmation

Biosafety level required for working with these viruses: BSL-4

Additional reading

Halpin K, Young PL, Field HE, Mackenzie JS. Isolation of Hendra virus from pteropid bats: a natural reservoir of Hendra virus. J Gen Virol 2000;81:1927–32.

Lamb RA, Kolakofsky D. Paramyxoviridae: the viruses and their replication. In: Knipe DM, Howley PM, editors. Fields virology. Vol 1. 4th ed. Philadelphia: Lippincott Williams & Wilkins; 2001. p. 1305–40.

Selvey LA, Wells RM, McCormack JG, et al. Infection of humans and horses by a newly described morbillivirus. Med J Aust 1995;162:642–5.

Williamson MM, Hooper PT, Selleck PW, et al. Transmission studies of Hendra virus (equine morbillivirus) in fruit bats, horses and cats. Aust Vet J 1998;76:813–8.

http://www.cdc.gov/ncidod/diseases/hendraq&a.htm (accessed September 21, 2002).

Herpes virus B infection
(Cercopithecine herpesvirus 1 infection, Herpes simiae virus infection)

Agent: herpes B virus, family Herpesviridae, genus *Simplexvirus* (DNA)

Reservoir: monkey, usually *Macaca* spp and cynomolgus

Vector: none

Vehicle: contact or bite

Incubation period: 10 d–20 d (range 2 d–60 d)

Clinical hints:

lymphadenopathy	myalgia
major neurological signs	singultus
monkey contact	skin vesicles

Typical therapy: Acyclovir 12.0 mg/kg IV q8h or Gancyclovir 5.0 mg/kg IV q12h; follow with prolonged Acyclovir 800 mg PO 5× daily

Disease distribution: precise distribution unknown

Notes

Herpes virus B was first isolated in 1933 from a fatal human case which followed a monkey bite.

The virus is often carried asymptomatically by Old World primates (rhesus *Macaca mulatta*, cynomolgus, *Macaca fascicularis*, *Macaca radiata*, *Macaca fasciata*, and *Macaca arctoides*). Latent viral infection among captive and feral macaques may approach 80 to 100%, with shedding in urogenital, conjunctival, and oral secretions.

The virus is present in buccal, conjunctival, and genital excreta of monkeys, particularly those that are ill, under stress, or breeding.

Human disease is acquired though bites or scratches; however, transmission has been documented among laboratory workers handling infected brain and kidney tissues and from material splashed into the eye.

Clinical presentation: Most human infections have been fatal, consisting of myelitis and hemorrhagic encephalitis with concomitant multi-organ involvement. The illness begins with fever, malaise, diffuse myalgia, nausea, abdominal pain, and headache, usually within 1 month following contact. Lymphadenitis is seen proximal to the site of inoculation. Neurologic findings then predominate, with dysesthesia, ataxia, diplopia, seizures, and ascending flaccid paralysis. Case-fatality rates exceed 80%. Lymphocytic cerebrospinal fluid pleocytosis and elevated protein levels are noted, often with numerous erythrocytes and elevated protein levels. In contrast to herpes simplex infection, the encephalitis is multifocal. Rarely, isolated skin infection, and even an isolated meningitis, may be encountered.

Specimens for diagnostic testing: material from lesions, serum

Patient isolation precautions: strict avoidance of contact with lesion material

Suggested assays for virus detection: detection of viral RNA by RT-PCR

Serodiagnosis: enzyme-linked immunosorbent assays for IgM and IgG antibodies

Biosafety level required for working with herpes virus B: BSL-4

Additional reading

Boulter EA, Thornton B, Bauer DJ, Bye A. Successful treatment of experimental B virus (Herpesvirus simiae) infection with acyclovir. Br Med J 1980;280:681–3.

Hartley EG. "B" virus: herpes virus simiae. Lancet 1966;1:87.

Holmes GP, Chapman LE, Stewart JA, et al. Guidelines for the prevention and treatment of B-virus infections in exposed persons. The B virus Working Group. Clin Infect Dis 1995;20:421–39.

Ostrowski SR, Leslie MJ, Parrott T, et al. B-virus from pet macaque monkeys: an emerging threat in the United States? Emerg Infect Dis 1998;4:117–21.

Whitley RJ, Hilliard JK. Cercopithecine herpesvirus (B virus). In: Knipe DM, Howley PM, editors. Fields virology. Vol 2. 4th ed. Philadelphia: Lippincott Williams & Wilkins; 2001. p. 2835–48.

http://research.ucsb.edu/connect/pro/disease.html#v4 (accessed September 21, 2002).

http://www.cdc.gov/epo/mmwr/preview/mmwrhtml/00015936.htm (accessed September 21, 2002).

and coma. In some cases, a sudden seizure is the presenting sign of disease. Nuchal rigidity and seizures are present in 50 to 75% of cases, and cranial nerve palsies in 33%. Other signs include hemiparesis, spastic paralysis, hyperreflexia, extrapyramidal signs, and abnormal reflexes. Evidence of increased intracranial pressure is relatively uncommon. Neurologic function is regained gradually over several weeks, with full recovery requiring months to years. The case-fatality rate in hospitals having intensive care facilities is 25%, and neurological residua are seen in 80% of patients.

Laboratory studies reveal peripheral leukocytosis with a left shift, and hyponatremia. CSF pleocytosis ranges from less than 10 to several thousand per cubic millimeter (usually hundreds). The CSF protein is typically normal or only mildly elevated.

Specimens for diagnostic testing: brain tissue, CSF, serum

Patient isolation precautions: prevent access by mosquitoes

Suggested assays for virus detection: detection of viral RNA by RT-PCR, virus isolation in cell cultures

Serodiagnosis: enzyme-linked immunosorbent assays for IgM and IgG antibodies, neutralization tests for confirmation

Biosafety level required for working with Japanese encephalitis virus: BSL-3

Additional reading

Anon. Japanese encephalitis vaccines. Wkly Epidemiol Rec 1998;73:337–44.

Burke DS, Monath TP. Flaviviruses. In: Knipe DM, Howley PM, editors. Fields virology. Vol 1. 4th ed. Philadelphia: Lippincott Williams & Wilkins; 2001. p. 1043–126.

Igarashi A. Epidemiology and control of Japanese encephalitis. World Health Stat Q 1992;45:299–305.

Lindenbach BD, Rice CM. Flaviviridae: the viruses and their replication. In: Knipe DM, Howley PM, editors. Fields virology. Vol 1. 4th ed. Philadelphia: Lippincott Williams & Wilkins; 2001. p. 991–1041.

Thompson RF, Bass DM, Hoffman SL. Travel vaccines. Infect Dis Clin North Am 1999;13:149–67.

http://www.cdc.gov/ncidod/dvbid/arbor/index.htm (accessed September 21, 2002).

http://www.cdc.gov/ncidod/diseases/list_mosquitoborne.htm (accessed September 21, 2002).

http://www.cdc.gov/ncidod/dvbid/jencephalitis/index.htm (accessed September 21, 2002).

Kyasanur Forest disease
(Monkey fever)

Agent: Kyasanur Forest disease virus, family Flaviviridae, genus *Flavivirus* (RNA)

Reservoir: rodent, shrew, monkey, bat, bird, tick

Vector: tick (*Haemaphysalis spinigera*, *Haemaphysalis turturis*, *Haemaphysalis papuana*)

Vehicle: none

Incubation period: 3 d–12 d

Clinical hints:

conjunctivitis	myalgia
encephalitis	palatal vesicles
generalized lymphadenopathy	relative bradycardia
history of tick bite	thrombocytopenia
leukopenia	vomiting

Typical therapy: symptomatic

Disease distribution: India

Notes

This disease was first described in 1957 in the Kyasanur Forest of Karnataka State, India.

Disease rates peak during the months of January and February.

Local reservoirs include black-faced langurs (*Presbytis entellus*), macaques (*Macaca radiata*), shrews (*Suncus murinus*), rats (*Rattus wroughtoni*), birds, squirrels, and bats. The appearance of dead monkeys in the endemic area may herald an epidemic.

In 1994, fatal infection by "**Fakeeh**" virus (= Alkhurma virus), now suspected to be a newly recognized flavivirus, was documented in Saudi Arabia. Illness was characterized by fever, rigors, hemorrhagic diatheses, morbilliform rash, encephalitis, leukopenia, thrombocytopenia, and hepatic and renal dysfunction. Several of the patients were foreigners, and had been in contact with sheep, beef, or camel meat or raw camel milk. Initial testing suggests that this virus is related to that of Kyasanur Forest disease.

In 2000, outbreaks were reported in Honnavar, Joida, and Siddapur, resulting in 9 deaths, of which 2 were virologically confirmed.

Clinical presentation: Clinical features and epidemiology of Kyasanur Forest disease are similar to those of other tick-borne flaviviruses. Illness begins abruptly with fever, headache, chills, vomiting, myalgia, photophobia, and conjunctivitis. Physical findings may include facial erythema, lymphadenopathy, hepatospenomegaly, and hemorrhagic phenomena such as petechiae, epistaxis, and gastrointestinal bleeding. Forty percent of patients develop hemorrhagic pulmonary edema, and renal failure is occasionally encountered. In 15 to 50% of patients, a second phase of illness follows a quiescent period of 1 to 3 weeks, and is characterized by neurologic symptoms. Laboratory findings include leukopenia, thrombocytopenia, hemoconcentration, and hepatic dysfunction.

Specimens for diagnostic testing: blood (not frozen), serum

Patient isolation precautions: strict containment

Suggested assays for virus detection: detection of viral RNA by RT-PCR, virus isolation not recommended

Serodiagnosis: enzyme-linked immunosorbent assays for IgM and IgG antibodies, neutralization tests for confirmation

Biosafety level required for working with Kyasanur Forest disease virus: BSL-4

Additional reading

Adhikari Prabha MR, Prabhu MG, Raghuveer CV, et al. Clinical study of 100 cases of Kyasanur Forest disease with clinicopathological correlation. Indian J Med Sci 1993;47:124–30.

Banerjee K. Emerging viral infections with special reference to India. Indian J Med Res 1996;103:177–200.

Boshell J. Kyasanur Forest disease: ecologic considerations. Am J Trop Med Hyg 1969;18:67–80.

Burke DS, Monath TP. Flaviviruses. In: Knipe DM, Howley PM, editors. Fields virology. Vol 1. 4th ed. Philadelphia: Lippincott Williams & Wilkins; 2001. p. 1043–126.

Lindenbach BD, Rice CM. Flaviviridae: the viruses and their replication. In: Knipe DM, Howley PM, editors. Fields virology. Vol 1. 4th ed. Philadelphia: Lippincott Williams & Wilkins; 2001. p. 991–1041.

Pavri K. Clinical, clinicopathologic, and hematologic features of Kyasanur Forest disease. Rev Infect Dis 1989;11 Suppl 4: S854–9.

Sreenivasan MA, Bhat HR, Rajagopalan PK. The epizootics of Kyasanur Forest disease in wild monkeys during 1964 to 1973. Trans R Soc Trop Med Hyg 1986;80:810–14.

Lassa fever

Agent: Lassa virus, family Arenaviridae, genus *Arenavirus* (RNA)

Reservoir: multimammate mouse (*Mastomys huberti, Mastomys erythroleucus, Mastomys natalensis*, and other rodents)

Vector: none

Vehicle: rodent secretions, dust, food, patient secretions

Incubation period: 8 d–14 d (range 3 d–21 d)

Clinical hints:

conjunctivitis	leukopenia
cough	pharyngitis
gastrointestinal symptoms	proteinuria
hepatic dysfunction	retrosternal pain

Typical therapy: strict isolation; Ribavirin 2.0 g IV, then 1.0 g IV q6h × 4 d, then 0.5 g IV q8h × 6 d

Disease distribution:

Burkina Faso	Mali
Central African Republic	Mozambique
Gabon	Nigeria
Gambia	Senegal
Ghana	Sierra Leone
Guinea	Uganda
Ivory Coast	Zimbabwe
Liberia	

Considered a potential bioterrorism weapon.

Notes

Lassa fever is thought to occur in all of West Africa, from Nigeria to Senegal. As many as 500,000 cases may occur yearly, according to some estimates. Disease rates peak during January to April, that is, the dry season. Twelve cases of Lassa fever were imported into Europe and North America during 1970 to 2000, with no secondary cases among medical staff or patients. Four cases were imported into Europe during January to July 2000.

The disease is transmitted to humans from wild rodents. Lassa infection persists in rodents and the virus is shed throughout the life of the animal. Disease transmission is primarily through direct or indirect contact with excreta of infected rodents deposited on surfaces such as floors, beds, or in food or water. All age groups are susceptible to Lassa virus infection. Person-to-person and laboratory infections occur, especially in the hospital environment, by direct contact with blood that includes inoculation with contaminated needles, pharyngeal secretions or urine, or by sexual contact. Person-to-person spread may occur during the acute phase of fever when the virus is present in the throat. The virus may be excreted in the urine of patients for 3 to 9 weeks from the onset of illness. The virus can be transmitted via semen for up to 3 months. Nosocomial outbreaks have been described in Nigeria, Liberia, and Sierra Leone.

Clinical presentation: The onset of symptoms is gradual, with fever, malaise, headache, sore throat, cough, nausea, vomiting, diarrhea, myalgia, and chest and abdominal pain. The fever may be either constant or intermittent with spikes. Inflammation of the throat and eyes is commonly observed. In severe cases, hypotension or shock, pleural effusion, hemorrhage, seizures, encephalopathy, and swelling of the face and neck are frequent. Approximately 15% of hospitalized cases do not survive. The disease is more severe in pregnancy, and fetal loss occurs in greater than 80% of cases. Hair loss and loss of coordination may occur in convalescence. Sensorineural deafness occurs in 29% of cases, making this the most common cause of deafness in West Africa.

The clinical syndrome of Lassa fever is difficult to distinguish from severe malaria, septicemia, yellow fever, and other viral hemorrhagic fevers such as Ebola fever. Inflammation of the throat with white tonsillar patches is an important distinguishing feature. Definitive diagnosis requires testing that is available only in highly specialized laboratories.

Specimens for diagnostic testing: serum, liver, spleen, throat washings, body fluids

Patient isolation precautions: strict isolation

Suggested assays for virus detection: detection of viral RNA by RT-PCR, virus isolation not recommended

Serodiagnosis: enzyme-linked immunosorbent assays and immunofluorescence assays for IgM and IgG antibodies

Biosafety level required for working with Lassa virus: BSL-4

Additional reading

Anon. Lassa fever. Update. Wkly Epidemiol Rec 1996;71:194.

Bajani MD, Tomori O, Rollin PE, et al. A survey for antibodies to Lassa virus among health workers in Nigeria. Trans R Soc Trop Med Hyg 1997;91:379–81.

Buchmeier MJ, Bowen MD, Peters CJ. Arenaviridae: the viruses and their replication. In: Knipe DM, Howley PM, editors. Fields virology. Vol 2. 4th ed. Philadelphia: Lippincott Williams & Wilkins; 2001. p. 1635–68.

Fisher-Hoch SP, Tomori O, Nasidi A, et al. Review of cases of nosocomial Lassa fever in Nigeria: the high price of poor medical practice. Br Med J 1995;311:857–9.

Frame JD. Clinical features of Lassa fever in Liberia. Rev Infect Dis 1989;11 Suppl 4:S783–9.

Johnson KM, Monath TP. Imported Lassa fever — reexamining the algorithms [editorial]. N Engl J Med 1990;323:1139–41.

McCormick JB, Webb PA, Krebs JW, et al. A prospective study of the epidemiology and ecology of Lassa fever. J Infect Dis 1987;155:437–44.

McCormick JB, King IJ, Webb PA, et al. Lassa fever. Effective therapy with ribavirin. N Engl J Med 1986;314:20–6.

Speed BR, Gerrard MP, Kennett ML, et al. Viral haemorrhagic fevers: current status, future threats. Med J Aust 1996;164:79–83.

http://www.who.int/emc/diseases/ebola/index.html (accessed September 21, 2002).

http://www.cdc.gov/ncidod/dvrd/spb/mnpages/dispages/arena.htm (accessed September 21, 2002).

http://www.emedicine.com/emerg/topic887.htm (accessed September 21, 2002).

Louping ill
(La tremblante du mouton, Ovine encephalomyelitis, Scottish sheep encephalomyelitis, Thwarter ill, Trembling ill)

Agent: louping ill virus, family Flaviviridae, genus *Flavivirus* (RNA)

Reservoir: tick, sheep, deer, grouse

Vector: tick (*Ixodes ricinus*)

Vehicle: dairy products

Incubation period: 4 d–7 d (range 1 d–8 d)

Clinical hints:

biphasic illness	leukocytosis
contact with sheep	meningitis
encephalitis	tick bite

Typical therapy: symptomatic

Disease distribution: Ireland, United Kingdom

Notes

Louping ill is a severe neurological disease of sheep that is occasionally transmitted to humans. Human infection by louping ill virus is confined to Great Britain; however, the virus has been demonstrated in sheep in Spain, and birds and horses in Ireland.

Highest tick (*Ixodes ricinus*) activity occurs in the spring and fall. Seventeen natural infections and 26 laboratory infections were reported in 1991. Eight percent of slaughterhouse workers in endemic areas are seropositive.

The principal reservoirs are sheep and red grouse (*Lagopus lagopus scoticus*). The virus has also been isolated from shrews (*Sorex araneus*) and field mice (*Apodemus sylvaticus*).

Clinical presentation: The disease is biphasic, beginning with fever, headache, photophobia, myalgia, arthralgia, leukopenia, and lymphadenopathy. The acute illness resolves within 1 month, and is followed by a second stage characterized by meningitis and leukocytosis. Recovery is complete; however, convalescence may be prolonged.

Specimens for diagnostic testing: blood, CSF, serum

Patient isolation precautions: none

Suggested assays for virus detection: detection of viral RNA by RT-PCR, virus isolation in cell cultures

Serodiagnosis: enzyme-linked immunosorbent assays for IgM and IgG antibodies, neutralization tests for confirmation

Biosafety level required for working with louping ill virus: BSL-3

Additional reading

Burke DS, Monath TP. Flaviviruses. In: Knipe DM, Howley PM, editors. Fields virology. Vol 1. 4th ed. Philadelphia: Lippincott Williams & Wilkins; 2001. p. 1043–126.

Davidson MM, Williams H, Macleod JA. Louping ill in man: a forgotten disease. J Infect 1991;23:241–9.

Lindenbach BD, Rice CM. Flaviviridae: the viruses and their replication. In: Knipe DM, Howley PM, editors. Fields virology. Vol 1. 4th ed. Philadelphia: Lippincott Williams & Wilkins; 2001. p. 991–1041.

Reid HW, Gibbs CA, Burrells C, Doherty PC. Laboratory infections with louping-ill virus. Lancet 1972;1:592–3.

Lymphocytic choriomeningitis

Agent: lymphocytic choriomeningitis virus, family Arenaviridae, genus *Arenavirus* (RNA)

Reservoir: house mouse, guinea pig, hamster, monkey

Vector: none

Vehicle: urine, saliva, feces, food, dust

Incubation period: 8 d–12 d (range 6 d–14 d)

Clinical hints:

encephalitis
exposure to rodents
headache
myalgia
meningitis
photophobia
pharyngitis

Typical therapy: symptomatic

Disease distribution: precise distribution unknown

Notes

Rodent infection by lymphocytic choriomeningitis virus occurs worldwide; however, human disease has only been described in Europe and the Americas. It is included in this book because it is an underreported disease.

The primary host is the house mouse (*Mus musculus* and *Mus domesticus*). Hamsters (*Mesocricetus auratus*) have also been implicated in some cases.

Clinical presentation: Thirty-five percent of infections are asymptomatic, and 50% are characterized by a nonspecific flu-like illness. Overt infections are characterized by fever, headache and systemic symptoms, leukopenia, and thrombocytopenia. Patients may also exhibit lymphadenopathy and a maculopapular rash, where 12 to 15% of patients have rash and/or meningitis or encephalitis. Relapses are characterized by a more severe headache, and meningitis may occur after initial improvement. Papilledema may be noted, and the CSF protein concentration ranges from 50 to 300 mg/dL, with a pleocytosis of several hundred lymphocytes/mm^3. Decreases in CSF glucose concentration are documented in more than 20% of cases.

Complications include encephalitis, psychosis, paraplegia, transitory aqueductal stenosis, and disturbances of cranial, sensory, or autonomic nervous function. Occasionally, orchitis, myocarditis, arthritis, or alopecia is encountered. Lymphocytic choriomeningitis is increasingly recognized as a cause of congenital chorioretinitis and blindness.

Specimens for diagnostic testing: serum, throat washings, CSF

Patient isolation precautions: none

Suggested assays for virus detection: detection of viral RNA by RT-PCR; virus isolation is difficult, but a convenient method is by inoculation of mouse foot pads

Serodiagnosis: enzyme-linked immunosorbent assays for IgM and IgG antibodies

Biosafety level required for working with lymphocytic choriomeningitis virus: BSL-3

Additional reading

Barton LL, Hyndman NJ. Lymphocytic choriomeningitis virus: a reemerging central nervous system pathogen. Pediatrics 2000;105:E35.

Buchmeier MJ, Bowen MD, Peters CJ. Arenaviridae: the viruses and their replication. In: Knipe DM, Howley PM, editors. Fields virology. Vol 2. 4th ed. Philadelphia: Lippincott Williams & Wilkins; 2001. p. 1635–68.

Enders G, Varho Gobel M, Lohler J, et al. Congenital lymphocytic choriomeningitis virus infection: an underdiagnosed disease. Pediatr Infect Dis J 1999;18:652–5.

Park JY, Peters CJ, Rollin PE, et al. Age distribution of lymphocytic choriomeningitis virus serum antibody in Birmingham, Alabama: evidence of a decreased risk of infection. Am J Trop Med Hyg 1997;57:37–41.

Rousseau MC, Saron MF, Brouqui P, Bourgeade A. Lymphocytic choriomeningitis virus in southern France: four case reports and a review of the literature. Eur J Epidemiol 1997;13:817–23.

Wright R, Johnson D, Neumann M, et al. Congenital lymphocytic choriomeningitis virus syndrome: a disease that mimics congenital toxoplasmosis or Cytomegalovirus infection. Pediatrics 1997;100:E9.

http://www.cdc.gov/ncidod/dvrd/spb/mnpages/dispages/arena.htm (accessed September 21, 2002).

http://www.cdc.gov/ncidod/dvrd/spb/mnpages/dispages/lcmv.htm (accessed September 21, 2002).

Marburg virus disease
(Durba syndrome, African green monkey disease)

Agent: Marburg virus, family Filoviridae, genus *Marburgvirus* (RNA)

Reservoir: African green monkey (*Cercopithecus aethiops*)

Vector: none

Vehicle: secretions, contact, syringe, needle

Incubation period: 5 d–7 d (range 3 d–13 d)

Clinical hints:

- arthralgia
- conjunctivitis
- contact with primate
- diarrhea
- fever
- hemorrhagic diatheses
- hepatic dysfunction
- maculopapular rash
- myalgia
- sore throat
- vomiting

Typical therapy: symptomatic

Disease distribution:

- Central African Republic
- Democratic Republic of Congo
- Gabon
- Kenya
- Liberia
- Nigeria
- South Africa
- Sudan
- Uganda
- Zimbabwe

Considered a potential bioterrorism weapon.

Notes

Marburg disease was first described in Marburg (Germany) and in the former Yugoslavia in 1967; 31 cases were associated with imported green monkeys (*C. aethiops*).

Two bat cave-associated cases were identified in Kenya in 1980 and 1987, with additional sporadic cases in Zimbabwe and South Africa.

The world's first extensive outbreak of Marburg fever occurred in the Democratic Republic of Congo during 1998 to 1999; additional cases occurred in the area in 2000.

Clinical presentation: The symptoms and signs of Marburg and Ebola virus infections are similar. Following an incubation period of 4 to 16 days, onset is sudden, marked by anorexia, fever, chills, headache, and myalgia. Later, the patient develops nausea, vomiting, sore throat, abdominal pain, and diarrhea. Patients are dehydrated, apathetic, and disoriented, and exhibit pharyngeal and conjunctival injection. Most develop severe hemorrhagic manifestations between days 5 and 7 after onset. Bleeding is often from multiple sites, most commonly from the gastrointestinal tract, lungs, and gingivae. Hemorrhage and oropharyngeal lesions carry a particularly poor prognosis. Orchitis, uveitis, and hearing loss may occur late in the illness. Death occurs between the seventh to sixteenth day of illness.

Specimens for diagnostic testing: blood, serum, liver, spleen

Patient isolation precautions: strict isolation

Suggested assays for virus detection: detection of viral RNA by RT-PCR, virus isolation not recommended

Serodiagnosis: enzyme-linked immunosorbent assays and immunofluorescence assays for IgM and IgG antibodies

Biosafety level required for working with Marburg virus: BSL-4

Additional reading

Anon. Marburg fever, Democratic Republic of the Congo. Wkly Epidemiol Rec 1999;74:145.

Feldmann H, Slenczka W, Klenk HD. Emerging and reemerging filoviruses. Arch Virol 1996;11 Suppl:77–100.

Gear JH. Clinical aspects of African viral hemorrhagic fevers. Rev Infect Dis 1989;11 Suppl 4:S777–82.

LeDuc JW. Epidemiology of hemorrhagic fever viruses. Rev Infect Dis 1989;11 Suppl 4:S730–5.

Monath TP. Ecology of Marburg and Ebola viruses: speculations and directions for future research. J Infect Dis 1999;179 Suppl 1:S127–38.

Sanchez A, Khan AS, Zaki SR, et al. Filoviridae: Marburg and Ebola viruses. In: Knipe DM, Howley PM, editors. Fields virology. Vol 1. 4th ed. Philadelphia: Lippincott Williams & Wilkins; 2001. p. 1279–304.

Slenczka WG. The Marburg virus outbreak of 1967 and subsequent episodes. Curr Top Microbiol Immunol 1999;235:49–75.

http://www.cdc.gov/ncidod/diseases/virlfvr/virlfvr.htm (accessed September 21, 2002).

http://www.emedicine.com/emerg/topic887.htm (accessed September 21, 2002).

Mayaro fever

Agent: Mayaro virus, family Togaviridae, genus *Alphavirus* (RNA)

Reservoir: possibly primate

Vector: mosquito (*Haemagogus janthinomys*)

Vehicle: none

Incubation period: 3 d–12 d

Clinical hints:

arthralgia	lymphadenopathy
forest exposure	maculopapular rash
headache	myalgia

Typical therapy: symptomatic

Disease distribution:

Bolivia	Guyana
Brazil	Panama
Colombia	Peru
Ecuador	Suriname
French Guiana	Trinidad & Tobago

Notes

Mayaro is an acute, self-limited, dengue-like illness limited to South America. The virus has also been found in a migratory bird arriving in Louisiana in the United States. The disease is named for Mayaro County, Trinidad, where the first isolation was made in 1954.

Outbreaks are described among new immigrants to endemic areas. As many as 60% of some groups of Amazonian Indians are seropositive.

Mosquito transmission of the Mayaro virus is highest during the afternoon. Wild vertebrates maintain the virus in nature, and the local vectors are *Haemagogus* spp mosquitoes. *Coquillettidia venezuelensis*, *Psorophora ferox*, and *Sabethini* spp have also been implicated.

Clinical presentation: Mayaro fever is characterized by abrupt onset of fever, chills, myalgia, and headache. Gastrointestinal symptoms may also be present, and lymphadenopathy is found in 50% of patients. Arthralgias of the small joints of hands and feet are present, and a maculopapular rash of the trunk and extremities appears on the second to fifth day of illness in two-thirds of patients. There are no sequelae; however, joint pain may persist for several months.

Specimens for diagnostic testing: blood, serum

Patient isolation precautions: prevent access by mosquitoes

Suggested assays for virus detection: detection of viral RNA by RT-PCR, virus isolation in cell cultures

Serodiagnosis: enzyme-linked immunosorbent assays for IgM and IgG antibodies, neutralization tests for confirmation

Biosafety level required for working with Mayaro virus: BSL-3

Additional reading

Griffin DE. Alphaviruses. In: Knipe DM, Howley PM, editors. Fields virology. Vol 1. 4th ed. Philadelphia: Lippincott Williams & Wilkins; 2001. p. 917–62.

Pinheiro FP, Freitas RB, Travassos da Rosa JF, et al. An outbreak of Mayaro virus disease in Belterra, Brazil. I. Clinical and virological findings. Am J Trop Med Hyg 1981;30:674–81.

Schlesinger S, Schlesinger MJ. Togaviridae: the viruses and

their replication. In: Knipe DM, Howley PM, editors. Fields virology. Vol 1. 4th ed. Philadelphia: Lippincott Williams & Wilkins; 2001. p. 895–916.

Talarmin A, Chandler LJ, Kazanji M, et al. Mayaro virus fever in French Guiana: isolation, identification, and seroprevalence. Am J Trop Med Hyg 1998;59:452–6.

Tesh RB, Watts DM, Russell KL, et al. Mayaro virus disease: an emerging mosquito-borne zoonosis in tropical South America. Clin Infect Dis 1999;28:67–73.

Monkeypox disease

Agent: monkeypox virus, family Poxviridae, genus *Orthopoxvirus* (DNA)

Reservoir: monkey, squirrel

Vector: none

Vehicle: contact

Incubation period: 10 d–12 d (range 7 d–20 d)

Clinical hints:

contact with a squirrel or monkey

painful lymphadenopathy
vesiculopustular rash

Typical therapy: symptomatic

Disease distribution:

Cameroon
Central African Republic
Democratic Republic of Congo
Gabon
Ivory Coast
Liberia
Nigeria
Sierra Leone

Considered a potential bioterrorism weapon.

Notes

Monkeypox was first recorded in monkeys in 1958, and in humans in 1970 (Zaire).

More than 800 cases have been registered, with the highest rates being among children. Most infections occur in areas of tropical rain forests during the dry season. Rare secondary cases are reported, most among family contacts. The attack rate among susceptible individuals is 10%. Prior smallpox vaccination appears to attenuate the severity of illness.

More than 500 cases were reported from the Democratic Republic of Congo during 1996 to 1997; and over 300 during 2000 to 2001.

Arboreal squirrels, such as Thomas' and Kuhl's tree squirrel (*Funisciurus* spp) and the sun squirrel (*Heliosciurus* spp), have been implicated as natural reservoirs.

Clinical presentation: Although clinical features of the disease resemble those of smallpox, most infections are mild. Typically, a papular rash with marked regional lymphadenopathy follows a 3-day prodrome, with most lesions appearing on the face and extremities including the palms and soles. Umbilicated pustules evolve, and leave a scar on healing. Infection resolves within 2 to 4 weeks. The case-fatality rate is 10 to 15%.

Specimens for diagnostic testing: vesicle fluid, serum

Patient isolation precautions: strict isolation

Suggested assays for virus detection: detection of viral RNA by RT-PCR, virus isolation in cell cultures

Serodiagnosis: enzyme-linked immunosorbent assays for IgM and IgG antibodies

Biosafety level required for working with monkeypox virus: BSL-2

Additional reading

Anon. Human monkeypox in Kasai Oriental, Democratic Republic of the Congo (former Zaire). Preliminary report of October 1997 investigation. Wkly Epidemiol Rec 1997;72: 369–72.

Breman JG, Henderson DA. Poxvirus dilemmas — monkeypox, smallpox, and biologic terrorism. N Engl J Med 1998;339: 556–9.

Esposito JJ, Fenner F. Poxviruses. In: Knipe DM, Howley PM, editors. Fields virology. Vol 2. 4th ed. Philadelphia: Lippincott Williams & Wilkins; 2001. p. 2885–921.

Heymann DL, Szczeniowski M, Esteves K. Re-emergence of monkeypox in Africa: a review of the past six years. Br Med Bull 1998;54:693–702.

Moss B. Poxviridae: the viruses and their replication. In: Knipe DM, Howley PM, editors. Fields virology. Vol 2. 4th ed. Philadelphia: Lippincott Williams & Wilkins; 2001. p. 2849–83.

Murray Valley encephalitis
(Australian X disease, Australian encephalitis)

Agent: Murray Valley encephalitis virus, family Flaviviridae, genus *Flavirirus* (RNA), a similar local disease is caused by Kunjin virus (a West Nile-like virus)

Reservoir: bird

Vector: mosquito (*Aedes normanensis*, *Culex annulirostris*, and *Culex bitaeniorhynchus*)

Vehicle: none

Incubation period: 5 d–15 d

Clinical hints:

headache	neurological signs
myalgia	photophobia

Typical therapy: symptomatic

Disease distribution:

Australia	Papua New Guinea
Indonesia	

Notes

Murray Valley encephalitis is found in Australia (Figure 6), with rare cases reported from Papua New Guinea.

Although overt infection is rare, severe and even fatal cases are reported.

Most cases occur during January to early May, with overt clinical disease being most common below the age of 15 and above the age of 50.

In 2001, nonfatal Murray Valley encephalitis was diagnosed in a German tourist who had visited Central and North-central Australia.

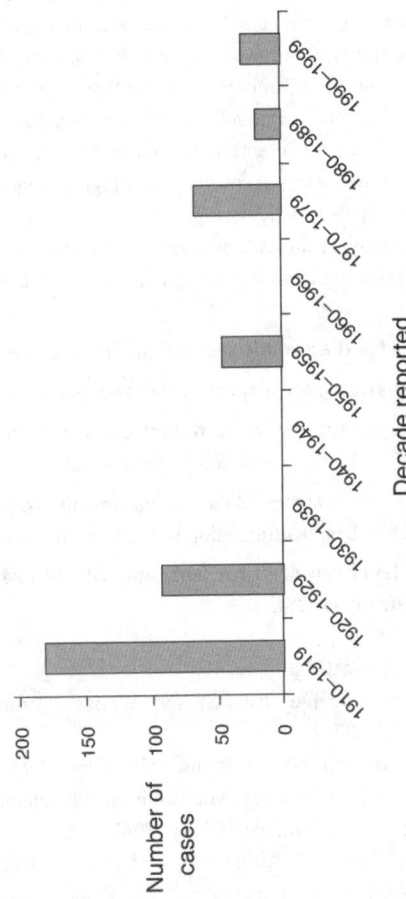

Figure 6 Murray Valley encephalitis in Australia.

Clinical presentation: Most cases occur during January through May. A prodrome of headache, vomiting, photophobia, and neck stiffness is followed within 2 to 5 days by changes in sensorium, stupor, and motor signs. Severe cases progress to coma, paralysis, and respiratory depression. Residual paralysis, motor disturbances, and emotional and psychologic symptoms are common following recovery. Neurological sequelae continue in over 30% of patients.

Diagnosis may be difficult because of the confusing presence of other flaviviruses causing similar illnesses, such as Kunjin virus.

Specimens for diagnostic testing: brain tissue, CSF, serum

Patient isolation precautions: prevent access by mosquitoes

Suggested assays for virus detection: detection of viral RNA by RT-PCR, virus isolation in cell cultures

Serodiagnosis: enzyme-linked immunosorbent assays for IgM and IgG antibodies, neutralization tests for confirmation

Biosafety level required for working with Murray Valley encephalitis virus: BSL-3

Additional reading

Anon. Communicable diseases surveillance. Commun Dis Intell 1997;21:107–15.

Burke DS, Monath TP. Flaviviruses. In: Knipe DM, Howley PM, editors. Fields virology. Vol 1. 4th ed. Philadelphia: Lippincott Williams & Wilkins; 2001. p. 1043–126.

Burrow JN, Whelan PI, Kilburn CJ, et al. Australian encephalitis in the Northern Territory: clinical and epidemiological features, 1987–1996. Aust N Z J Med 1998;28:590–6.

Lindenbach BD, Rice CM. *Flaviviridae*: the viruses and their replication. In: Knipe DM, Howley PM, editors. Fields virology. Vol 1. 4th ed. Philadelphia: Lippincott Williams & Wilkins; 2001. p. 991–1041.

Mackenzie JS, Lindsay MD, Coelen RJ, et al. Arboviruses causing human disease in the Australasian zoogeographic region. Arch Virol 1994;136:447–67.

Mackenzie JS, Smith DW, Broom AK, Bucens MR. Australian encephalitis in Western Australia, 1978–1991. Med J Aust 1993;158:591–5.

Russell RC. Mosquito-borne arboviruses in Australia: the current scene and implications of climate change for human health. Int J Parasitol 1998;28:955–69.

New World sandfly fevers

Agent: any of a number of viruses of the family Bunyaviridae, genus *Phlebovirus* (RNA)
Reservoir: possibly rodents
Vector: fly (sandfly: *Lutzomyia* spp)
Vehicle: none
Incubation period: 3 d–4 d (range 2 d–9 d)
Clinical hints:

arthralgia	no sequelae or fatality
eye pain	myalgia
facial flush	vomiting
leukopenia	

Typical therapy: symptomatic
Disease distribution:

Brazil	Panama
Colombia	

Considered a potential bioterrorism weapon.

Notes

The incidence of New World phlebovirus infection is unknown.

Sporadic cases or documented seroprevalence have been reported in Brazil (**Alenquer**, **Bujaru**, and **Candiru** viruses), Colombia (**Arboledas** and **Chagres** viruses), and Panama (**Cacao**, **Chagres**, **Changuinola**, and **Punta Toro** viruses).

Lutzomyia spp are the vectors for Arboledas, *Lutzomyia trapidoi* for Cacao, and *Lu. trapidoi* and *Lutzomyia ylephiletor* for Chagres and Punta Toro viruses.

Clinical presentation: Sandfly fevers usually begin abruptly with fever, and are associated with severe frontal headache, retro-orbital pain, photophobia, conjuctival injection, and back pain. The disease is self-limited in 2 to 3 days.

Specimens for diagnostic testing: serum, CSF, brain tissue

Patient isolation precautions: prevent access by arthropods

Suggested assays for virus detection: detection of viral RNA by RT-PCR, virus isolation in cell cultures

Serodiagnosis: enzyme-linked immunosorbent assays for IgM and IgG antibodies, neutralization tests for confirmation

Biosafety level required for working with these phleboviruses: BSL-3

Additional reading

Nichol ST. Bunyaviruses. In: Knipe DM, Howley PM, editors. Fields virology. Vol 2. 4th ed. Philadelphia: Lippincott Williams & Wilkins; 2001. p. 1603–33.

Schmaljohn CS, Hooper JW. Bunyaviridae: the viruses and their replication. In: Knipe DM, Howley PM, editors. Fields virology. Vol 2. 4th ed. Philadelphia: Lippincott Williams & Wilkins; 2001. p. 1581–602.

Srihongse S, Johnson CM. Human infections with Chagres virus in Panama. Am J Trop Med Hyg 1974;23:690–3.

Tesh RB, Boshell J, Young DG, et al. Biology of Arboledas virus, a new phlebotomus fever serogroup virus (Bunyaviridae: *Phlebovirus*) isolated from sand flies in Colombia. Am J Trop Med Hyg 1986;35:1310–6.

Travassos da Rosa AP, Tesh RB, Pinheiro FP, et al. Characterization of eight new phlebotomus fever serogroup arboviruses (Bunyaviridae: *Phlebovirus*) from the Amazon region of Brazil. Am J Trop Med Hyg 1983;32:1164–71.

Nipah virus disease

Agent: Nipah virus, family Paramyxoviridae, genus not yet assigned (RNA)

Reservoir: bats

Vector: unknown

Vehicle: unknown, possibly urine and secretions

Incubation period: unknown

Clinical hints:

contact with pigs	headache
coma	meningismus
encephalopathy	myoclonus
fever	

Typical therapy: symptomatic

Disease distribution: Bangladesh, Malaysia, Singapore

Notes

Nipah virus, named for Baru Sungai Nipa village in Malaysia, was implicated in at least 200 cases of encephalitis in Malaysia, occurring in Perak (Kinta) and Negri Sembilan (Sikamat and Bukit Pelandok) during 1998 to 1999. Eleven additional cases were reported in Singapore at the time.

Various species of fruit bats (*Pteropus* spp) are thought to serve as the natural reservoirs of the virus, with pigs as amplifying hosts. Antibody to the virus is also found in dogs, cats, horses, goats, and bats, including bats consumed by humans in certain parts of the world. The presumed vehicles are body secretions, possibly including urine.

Although contact with live pigs is the major factor in transmission, persons handling raw pork are at minimal risk.

An outbreak of encephalitis in Bangladesh during 2001 was ascribed to Nipah-like virus. Additional Nipah-related viruses have been isolated from fruit bats in Malaysia.

Nipah virus is considered a potential bioterrorism weapon.

Clinical presentation: The disease follows contact with blood from infected pigs. The illness is characterized by 3 to 14 days of fever, vomiting, headache, and drowsiness, progressing to coma within 24 to 48 hours. Segmental myoclonus, areflexia, hypotonia, hypertension, and tachycardia are common. The case-fatality rate is 32%. The illness in pigs is characterized by labored breathing, "Mile-long" cough, lethargy, and aggressive behavior.

Specimens for diagnostic testing: brain tissue, urine, CSF, serum

Patient isolation precautions: routine

Suggested assays for virus detection: detection of viral RNA by RT-PCR, virus isolation in cell cultures

Serodiagnosis: enzyme-linked immunosorbent assays for IgM and IgG antibodies, neutralization tests for confirmation

Biosafety level required for working with Nipah and closely-related viruses: BSL-4

Additional reading

Chew MH, Arguin PM, Shay DK, et al. Risk factors for Nipah virus infection among abattoir workers in Singapore. J Infect Dis 2000;181:1760–3.

Chua KB, Bellini WJ, Rota PA, et al. Nipah virus: a recently emergent deadly paramyxovirus. Science 2000;288:1432–5.

Goh KJ, Tan CT, Chew NK, et al. Clinical features of Nipah virus encephalitis among pig farmers in Malaysia. N Engl J Med 2000;342:1229–35.

Lamb RA, Kolakofsky D. Paramyxoviridae: the viruses and their replication. In: Knipe DM, Howley PM, editors. Fields virology. Vol 1. 4th ed. Philadelphia: Lippincott Williams & Wilkins; 2001. p. 1305–40.

Parashar UD, Sunn LM, Ong F, et al. Case-control study of risk factors for human infection with a new zoonotic paramyxovirus, Nipah virus, during a 1998–1999 outbreak of severe encephalitis in Malaysia. J Infect Dis 2000;181:1755–9.

Old World sandfly fevers
(Naples sandfly fever, Sicilian sandfly fever, Pappataci fever, Phlebotomus fever)

Agent: any of many viruses in the Phlebotomus fever serogroup, family Bunyaviridae, genus *Phlebovirus* (RNA)

Reservoir: rodents

Vector: fly (sandfly: *Phlebotomus papatasi* for Naples and Sicilian, *Phlebotomus perfilewi* for Naples)

Vehicle: none

Incubation period: 3 d–4 d (range 2 d–9 d)

Clinical hints:

arthralgia	leukopenia
eye pain	myalgia
facial flush	vomiting

Typical therapy: symptomatic

Disease distribution:

Afghanistan	India
Albania	Iran
Algeria	Iraq
Bahrain	Israel
Bangladesh	Italy
Bulgaria	Jordan
Canary Islands	Kuwait
China	Lebanon
Cyprus	Libya
Egypt	Malta
Ethiopia	Mauritania
Gibraltar	Monaco
Greece	Morocco

Nepal	Somalia
Oman	Spain
Pakistan	Sudan
Portugal	Tunisia
Qatar	Turkey
Russia (former Soviet Union)	Yemen
	Yugoslavia (former)
Saudi Arabia	

Considered a potential bioterrorism weapon.

Notes

During World War II, 19,000 military personnel developed sandfly fever, most in the Middle East.

Two distinct serotypes are found; **Sicilian** virus and **Naples** virus. A third, **Toscana** virus, is the only neurotropic virus transmitted by sandflies.

Highest rates are registered during April to October in the Mediterranean basin, the Middle East, India, Iran, the Caucasus, and Pakistan.

Sporadic cases have been described along the western coast of Saudi Arabia and in much of Iraq.

High attack rates occur among military personnel entering from nonendemic areas.

Highest rates are reported during summer in temperate regions.

Clinical presentation: Most infections are characterized by abrupt onset of fever, frontal headache, generalized myalgia, back pain, conjunctivitis, eye pain, photophobia, and prominent neutropenia. Vomiting, vertigo, and stiff neck have been described in some cases. Patients recover completely within 1 to 2 weeks. Neither sequelae nor fatal cases have been reported.

Specimens for diagnostic testing: blood, serum, CSF

Patient isolation precautions: prevent access by arthropods

Suggested assays for virus detection: detection of viral RNA by RT-PCR, virus isolation in cell cultures

Serodiagnosis: enzyme-linked immunosorbent assays for IgM and IgG antibodies, neutralization tests for confirmation

Biosafety level required for working with these phleboviruses: BSL-3

Additional reading

Bartelloni PJ, Tesh RB. Clinical and serologic responses of volunteers infected with phlebotomus fever virus (Sicilian type). Am J Trop Med Hyg 1976;25:456–62.

Calisher CH, Weinberg AN, Muth DJ, Lazuick JS. Toscana virus infection in a United States citizen returning from Italy. Lancet 1987;17:165–6.

Nichol ST. Bunyaviruses. In: Knipe DM, Howley PM, editors. Fields virology. Vol 2. 4th ed. Philadelphia: Lippincott Williams & Wilkins; 2001. p. 1603–33.

Nicoletti L, Ciufolini MG, Verani P. Sandfly fever viruses in Italy. Arch Virol 1996;11 Suppl:41–7.

Schmaljohn CS, Hooper JW. Bunyaviridae: the viruses and their replication. In: Knipe DM, Howley PM, editors. Fields virology. Vol 2. 4th ed. Philadelphia: Lippincott Williams & Wilkins; 2001. p. 1581–602.

Tesh RB. The epidemiology of Phlebotomus (sandfly) fever. Isr J Med Sci 1989;25:214–7.

Tesh RB, Saidi S, Gajdamovic SJ, et al. Serological studies on the epidemiology of sandfly fever in the Old World. Bull World Health Organ 1976;54:663–74.

Omsk hemorrhagic fever
(Muskrat fever, Spring-Autumn fever)

Agent: Omsk hemorrhagic fever virus, family Flaviviridae, genus *Flavivirus* (RNA)

Reservoir: rodents, muskrats (*Ondrata zibethica*), ticks

Vector: tick (*Dermacentor pictus* and *Dermacentor marginatus*)

Vehicle: none

Incubation period: 3 d–9 d (range 2 d–12 d)

Clinical hints:

gastrointestinal symptoms
headache
history of tick or muskrat contact
leukopenia
meningitis
myalgia
pulmonary symptoms
bleeding diathesis

Typical therapy: symptomatic

Disease distribution:

Romania

Russian Republic (northwestern Siberia — Omsk, Tyumen, Novosibirsk, and Kurgan regions)

Considered a potential bioterrorism weapon.

Notes

Omsk hemorrhagic fever was first reported during an outbreak in the Omsk district from 1943 to 1944. The virus was first isolated in 1947.

Disease incidence peaks in April to June, and September to November, and is limited to western and northwestern Siberia.

Cases during winter are associated with hunting activities. Most patients are rural residents, hunters, and agricultural workers.

Novosibirsk Region reported no cases from 1962 to 1987. There were 22 cases in 1989, 29 in 1990, 41 in 1991, 7 in 1992, 19 in 1993, 11 in 1994, 5 in 1995, 2 in 1996, and 7 in 1998 of which one was fatal.

The local vectors are *D. pictus* (north) and *D. marginatus* (south).

Clinical presentation: The onset of illness is abrupt, with fever, headache, myalgia, nausea, facial flushing, and a papulovesicular enanthem of the soft palate, progressing to hemorrhage from multiple mucosal surfaces. A biphasic fever course is noted in 30 to 50% of cases, with meningitis, renal dysfunction, or pneumonia during the second stage. Gastrointestinal symptoms, cough, relative bradycardia, leukopenia, thrombocytopenia, and lymphadenopathy are common, as are such sequelae as alopecia and hearing loss. The case-fatality rate is 0.5 to 2.5%.

Specimens for diagnostic testing: blood, serum

Patient isolation precautions: routine

Suggested assays for virus detection: detection of viral RNA by RT-PCR, virus isolation in suckling mice and cell cultures

Serodiagnosis: enzyme-linked immunosorbent assays for IgM and IgG antibodies, neutralization tests for confirmation

Biosafety level required for working with Omsk hemorrhagic fever virus: BSL-4

Additional reading

Anon. Viral haemorrhagic fevers. Report of a WHO Expert Committee. World Health Organ Tech Rep Ser 1985;721:5–126.
Burke DS, Monath TP. Flaviviruses. In: Knipe DM, Howley PM, editors. Fields virology. Vol 1. 4th ed. Philadelphia: Lippincott Williams & Wilkins; 2001. p. 1043–126.

Kharitonova NN, Leonov YA. Omsk hemorrhagic fever. New Delhi: Oxonian Press Pvt Ltd; 1985. p. 230.

Lindenbach BD, Rice CM. Flaviviridae: the viruses and their replication. In: Knipe DM, Howley PM, editors. Fields virology. Vol 1. 4th ed. Philadelphia: Lippincott Williams & Wilkins; 2001. p. 991–1041.

Simpson DI. Viral hemorrhagic fevers in man. Bull World Health Organ 1979;57:19–32.

O'nyong-nyong fever

Agent: O'nyong-nyong virus, family Togaviridae, genus *Alphavirus* (RNA)

Reservoir: unknown

Vector: mosquito (*Anopheles funestus* and *Anopheles gambiae*)

Vehicle: none

Incubation period: 3 d–12 d

Clinical hints:

- cervical lymphadenopathy
- conjunctivitis
- leukopenia
- maculopapular rash
- myalgia
- pruritis
- severe arthralgia

Typical therapy: symptomatic

Disease distribution:

- Central African Republic
- Democratic Republic of Congo
- Ghana
- Ivory Coast
- Kenya
- Malawi
- Mozambique
- Nigeria
- Senegal
- Sierra Leone
- Sudan
- Tanzania
- Uganda

Notes

O'nyong-nyong means "weakening of the joints" in the Acholi dialect. The virus was first isolated in 1959 during an epidemic in Acholi, Uganda. Several million subsequent cases were reported in Uganda, Kenya, Tanzania, Malawi, and Mozambique between 1959 and 1961.

The virus was not subsequently isolated until 1978. A rural epidemic due to the related **Igbo Ora** virus was reported from the Ivory Coast during 1984 to 1985.

An outbreak beginning in June 1996 involved southwest Uganda (Mbarara, Masaka, Kabarole, and Rakai districts), spreading to northern Tanzania (Bukuba District). In 1997, the Ugandan epidemic continued to spread northwestward into the Sembabule area.

Clinical presentation: The disease is characterized by fever, arthralgia, headache, conjunctivitis, myalgia, and lymphadenopathy. The knees and ankles are most commonly involved, and lymphadenopathy affects primarily the cervical region. Most patients develop a generalized rash that may be pruritic. Fever resolves within 7 days; however, arthralgia may persist.

Specimens for diagnostic testing: blood, serum

Patient isolation precautions: prevent access by mosquitoes

Suggested assays for virus detection: detection of viral RNA by RT-PCR, virus isolation in suckling mice and cell cultures

Serodiagnosis: enzyme-linked immunosorbent assays for IgM and IgG antibodies, neutralization tests for confirmation

Biosafety level required for working with O'nyong-nyong virus: BSL-2

Additional reading

Griffin DE. Alphaviruses. In: Knipe DM, Howley PM, editors. Fields virology. Vol 1. 4th ed. Philadelphia: Lippincott Williams & Wilkins; 2001. p. 917–62.

Kiwanuka N, Sanders EJ, Rwaguma EB, et al. O'nyong-nyong fever in south-central Uganda, 1996–1997: clinical features and validation of a clinical case definition for surveillance purposes. Clin Infect Dis 1999;29:1243–50.

Powers AM, Brault AC, Tesh RB, Weaver SC. Re-emergence of Chikungunya and O'nyong-nyong viruses: evidence for distinct geographical lineages and distant evolutionary relationships. J Gen Virol 2000;81(Pt 2):471–9.

Sanders EJ, Rwaguma EB, Kawamata J, et al. O'nyong-nyong fever in south-central Uganda, 1996–1997: description of the epidemic and results of a household-based seroprevalence survey. J Infect Dis 1999;180:1436–43.

Schlesinger S, Schlesinger MJ. Togaviridae: the viruses and their replication. In: Knipe DM, Howley PM, editors. Fields virology. Vol 1. 4th ed. Philadelphia: Lippincott Williams & Wilkins; 2001. p. 895–916.

Orf virus disease
(Contagious pustular dermatitis, Ecthyma contagiosum, Ovine pustular dermatitis)

Agent: Orf virus, family Poxviridae, genus *Parapoxvirus* (DNA)

Reservoir: sheep, goat, reindeer, musk ox

Vector: none

Vehicle: contact, secretions, fomites

Incubation period: 3 d–6 d (range 2 d–7 d)

Clinical hints:

contact with sheep or goats usually limited to finger
dermal pustule or ulcer or hand
heals without scaring

Typical therapy: symptomatic

Disease distribution: precise distribution unknown

Notes

Orf virus disease is primarily a disease of sheep and goats, worldwide. Humans acquire infection through direct contact with infected oral mucosa or skin.

Clinical presentation: Human infection is milder than that of sheep, and usually limited to indolent vesicles and pustules on the hands. Pustules may attain a size of 1 to 2 cm, and are often associated with low-grade fever and regional lymphadenitis. Lesions heal over a period of 2 to 6 weeks, without scarring. Secondary bacterial infection, disseminated orf virus disease, and erythema multiforme have been described in some cases.

Specimens for diagnostic testing: skin biopsy or exudate

Patient isolation precautions: prevent contact with infected lesions and exudates

Suggested assays for virus detection: detection of viral nucleic acid by RT-PCR, virus isolation in cell cultures

Serodiagnosis: enzyme-linked immunosorbent assays for IgM and IgG antibodies, neutralization tests for confirmation

Biosafety level required for working with Orf virus: BSL-3

Additional reading

Bassioukas K, Orfanidou A, Stergiopoulou CH, Hatzis J. Orf. Clinical and epidemiological study. Australas J Dermatol 1993;34:119–23.

Buchan J. Characteristics of orf in a farming community in mid-Wales. Br Med J 1996;313:203–4.

Esposito JJ, Fenner F. Poxviruses. In: Knipe DM, Howley PM, editors. Fields virology. Vol 2. 4th ed. Philadelphia: Lippincott Williams & Wilkins; 2001. p. 2885–921.

Lo C, Mathisen G. Human orf in Los Angeles County. West J Med 1996;164:77–8.

Moss B. Poxviridae: the viruses and their replication. In: Knipe DM, Howley PM, editors. Fields virology. Vol 2. 4th ed. Philadelphia: Lippincott Williams & Wilkins; 2001. p. 2849–83.

Paiba GA, Thomas DR, Morgan KL, et al. Orf (contagious pustular dermatitis) in farmworkers: prevalence and risk factors in three areas of England. Vet Rec 1999;145:7–11.

Roingeard P, Machet L. Images in clinical medicine. Orf skin ulcer. N Engl J Med 1997;337:1131.

Oropouche fever

Agent: Oropouche virus, family Bunyaviridae, genus *Orthobunyavirus* (RNA), Simbu group

Reservoir: unknown

Vector: midge (*Culicoides paraensis*), mosquito (*Culex quinquefasciatus*, *Aedes serratus*, *Coquillettidia venezuelensis*)

Vehicle: none

Incubation period: 4 d–8 d (range 3 d–12 d)

Clinical hints:

arthralgia	leukopenia
gastrointestinal symptoms	myalgia
headache	

Typical therapy: symptomatic

Disease distribution:

Brazil	Peru
Colombia	Trinidad & Tobago
Panama	

Notes

Oropouche virus was first isolated from a forest worker in Trinidad in 1955.

The first epidemic was reported in Belem (Brazil) in 1961. The virus has since caused at least 27 epidemics in rural and urban communities of Brazil, Panama, and Peru.

In most outbreaks, all ages and both sexes have been equally prone to infection.

In addition to humans, the virus has been found in sloths (*Bradypus tridactylus*) and species of *Mansonia*, *Aedes*, *Culex*, and *Culicoides*.

The principal vector appears to be the midge (*C. paraensis*).

Clinical presentation: Oropouche fever is characterized by abrupt onset of fever, chills, myalgia, arthralgia, headache, photophobia, and leukopenia. A rash is present in 5% of cases, and meningitis in 4%. The disease lasts for 5 to 7 days. No fatal infections have been reported; however, relapses and prolonged convalescence are common.

Specimens for diagnostic testing: blood, CSF, serum

Patient isolation precautions: avoid access by insects

Suggested assays for virus detection: virus isolation in cell cultures

Serodiagnosis: enzyme-linked immunosorbent assays and immunofluorescence assays for IgM and IgG antibodies, neutralization tests for confirmation

Biosafety level required for working with Oropouche virus: BSL-3

Additional reading

Baisley KJ, Watts DM, Munstermann LE, Wilson ML. Epidemiology of endemic Oropouche virus transmission in upper Amazonian Peru. Am J Trop Med Hyg 1998;59:710–6.

LeDuc JW, Hoch AL, Pinheiro FP, da Rosa AP. Epidemic Oropouche virus disease in northern Brazil. Bull Pan Am Health Organ 1981;15:97–103.

Nichol ST. Bunyaviruses. In: Knipe DM, Howley PM, editors. Fields virology. Vol 2. 4th ed. Philadelphia: Lippincott Williams & Wilkins; 2001. p. 1603–33.

Pinheiro FP, Travassos da Rosa AP, Travassos da Rosa JF, et al. Oropouche virus. I. A review of clinical, epidemiological, and ecological findings. Am J Trop Med Hyg 1981;30:149–60.

Schmaljohn CS, Hooper JW. Bunyaviridae: the viruses and their replication. In: Knipe DM, Howley PM, editors. Fields virology. Vol 2. 4th ed. Philadelphia: Lippincott Williams & Wilkins; 2001. p. 1581–602.

Tesh RB. The emerging epidemiology of Venezuelan hemorrhagic fever and Oropouche fever in tropical South America. Ann NY Acad Sci 1994;740:129–37.

Powassan encephalitis

Agent: Powassan virus, family Flaviviridae, genus *Flavivirus* (RNA)

Reservoir: tick (*Ixodes* spp, *Dermacentor andersoni*), rodent (woodchuck), carnivore

Vector: tick (*Ixodes cookei*, *Ixodes marxi*, *Ixodes scapularis*; *Dermacentor andersoni* may also be involved in the United States)

Vehicle: dairy products (rare)

Incubation period: median 19 d (range 4 d–30 d)

Clinical hints:

fever	headache
focal neurological signs	history of tick bite

Typical therapy:

Disease distribution:

Canada	United States
Russian Republic	

Notes

Powassan virus was first isolated from a child with encephalitis in Powassan, Ontario, Canada in 1958.

Human infection has only been described in the United States, Canada, and the Russian Republic. No cases were reported from 1978 to 1994. A single case was reported from Massachusetts in 1995, one from Vermont in 1999, two from Maine in 2000, and another from Maine in 2001.

Antibody is also found in local squirrels, chipmunks, groundhogs, and foxes.

A focus has been found among *Ix. scapularis* (formerly *dammini*) ticks in Wisconsin, USA.

Clinical presentation: Most infections are asymptomatic, as reflected by high seropositivity rates in endemic areas. Overt infection is associated with focal neurological findings in more than 50% of cases. Only 50% of patients recall a tick bite. Signs and symptoms reported have included olfactory hallucinations, temporal lobe seizures, residual hemi- or quadriplegia, aphasia, and spinal paralysis with residual muscular wasting. The case-fatality rate is 20%. Permanent neurological sequelae are reported in 50% of cases.

The peripheral blood discloses leukopenia initially, leukocytosis up to 20,000/mm^3 during the second phase, and leukopenia prior to recovery. Thrombocytopenia and hepatic dysfunction have also been reported. A CSF pleocytosis of less than 100/mm^3 is characteristic, with lymphocytes predominating by the ninth day of illness. CSF protein levels may be initially normal, but rise over a period of weeks.

Specimens for diagnostic testing: brain tissue, CSF, serum

Patient isolation precautions: none

Suggested assays for virus detection: detection of viral RNA by RT-PCR, virus isolation in cell cultures

Serodiagnosis: enzyme-linked immunosorbent assays and immunofluorescence assays for IgM and IgG antibodies, neutralization tests for confirmation

Biosafety level required for working with Powassan virus: BSL-3

Additional reading

Anon. Arboviral disease — United States, 1994. MMWR Morb Mort Wkly Rep 1995;44:641–4.

Calisher CH. Medically important arboviruses of the United States and Canada. Clin Microbiol Rev 1994;7:89–116.

Embil JA, Camfield P, Artsob H, Chase DP. Powassan virus encephalitis resembling herpes simplex encephalitis. Arch Intern Med 1983;143:341–3.

Gholam BI, Puksa S, Provias JP. Powassan encephalitis: a case report with neuropathology and literature review. Can Med Assoc J 1999;161:419–42.

Kolski H, Ford Jones EL, Richardson S, et al. Etiology of acute childhood encephalitis at The Hospital for Sick Children, Toronto, 1994–1995. Clin Infect Dis 1998;26:398–409.

Pseudocowpox disease
(Milker's nodule)

Agent: pseudocowpox virus, family Poxviridae, genus *Parapoxvirus* (DNA)

Reservoir: cattle

Vector: none

Vehicle: contact

Incubation period: 5 d–14 d

Clinical hints:

contact with cattle	umbilicated nodule
mild regional lymphadenopathy	usually on the hand

Typical therapy: symptomatic

Disease distribution: precise distribution unknown

Notes

Pseudocowpox is found worldwide among persons working with dairy cattle.

Infection is common in cattle, and infects humans through direct contact with udders.

Clinical presentation: The clinical course is mild and self-limited, and characterized by a red-to-blue nodule associated with minimal lymphadenopathy. Note that the lymphadenopathy of cowpox is more overt and painful.

Specimens for diagnostic testing: skin biopsy or exudate

Patient isolation precautions: avoid contact with lesions

Suggested assays for virus detection: detection of viral nucleic acid by RT-PCR, virus isolation in cell cultures

Serodiagnosis: enzyme-linked immunosorbent assays for IgM and IgG antibodies, neutralization tests for confirmation

Biosafety level required for working with pseudocowpox virus: BSL-3

Additional reading

Esposito JJ, Fenner F. Poxviruses. In: Knipe DM, Howley PM, editors. Fields virology. Vol 2. 4th ed. Philadelphia: Lippincott Williams & Wilkins; 2001. p. 2885–921.

Hunt E. Infectious skin diseases of cattle. Vet Clin North Am Large Anim Pract 1984;6:155–74.

Moss B. Poxviridae: the viruses and their replication. In: Knipe DM, Howley PM, editors. Fields virology. Vol 2. 4th ed. Philadelphia: Lippincott Williams & Wilkins; 2001. p. 2849–83.

Fowler JR. Viral infections. Hand Clin 1989;5:613–27.

Rift Valley fever
(Enzootic hepatitis, Zinga)

Agent: Rift Valley fever virus, family Bunyaviridae, genus *Phlebovirus* (RNA)

Reservoir: ruminants

Vector: mosquito (*Culex*, *Aedes*, *Anopheles*, *Eretmapodites*, *Mansonia*, *Culicoides*, *Coquillettidia* spp)

Vehicle: none

Incubation period: 3 d–5 d (range 2 d–7 d)

Clinical hints:

arthralgia	maculopapular rash
contact with sheep or cattle	myalgia
headache	photophobia
jaundice	retinitis
	bleeding diathesis

Typical therapy: symptomatic

Angola	Madagascar
Botswana	Malawi
Burundi	Mali
Cameroon	Mauritania
Central African Republic	Mozambique
Chad	Namibia
Djibouti	Niger
Egypt	Nigeria
Ethiopia	Rwanda
Gabon	Saudi Arabia
Guinea	Senegal
Kenya	Somalia
Lesotho	South Africa

Sudan	Yemen
Swaziland	Zambia
Tanzania	Zimbabwe
Uganda	

Disease distribution:

Considered a potential bioterrorism weapon.

Notes

Rift Valley fever virus was first isolated during an outbreak among sheep in the Rift Valley, Kenya, in 1931.

An outbreak in Egypt during 1977 to 1978 involved 18,000 human cases, of which 598 were fatal. An outbreak in Kenya, Somalia, and Tanzania during 1997 to 1998 involved an estimated 89,000 humans.

The disease was first reported in West Africa in 1974, in mosquitoes in Senegal; however, large outbreaks in the area were not reported prior to an epidemic in southern Mauritania in 1987. The first outbreak outside of sub-Saharan Africa occurred in Egypt in 1977; serological surveys indicate that the virus had not been in Egypt prior to that year. Rift Valley fever was first reported outside of the African continent, in Saudi Arabia and Yemen, in 2000.

During epizootics, disease usually occurs first in animals, then in humans. Humans are infected either through mosquito bites, or through contact with the body fluids or organs of infected animals; infection is also possibly by aerosol or by ingestion of contaminated milk. Human infection occurs mainly among farmers and others at occupational risk. Sheep are more susceptible than cattle; goats are least susceptible. Outbreaks are often heralded by outbreaks of unexplained abortion amongst livestock. Infected bats have been identified in Guinea.

Vectors include *Eretmapodites chrysogaster*, *Aedes caballus*, *Aedes circumluteolus*, *Aedes lineatopennis*, *Aedes cumminsii* (Burkina Faso), *Culex theileri*, *Culex antennatus* (Nigeria), *Mansonia africana*, *Mansonia uniformis* (Burkina Faso), and *Culicoides* spp.

Interepizootic vectors belong to the *Aedes* subgenera *Neomelanoconion* in East Africa, *Aedimorphus* in West Africa, and *Cx. theileri* in South Africa; *Aedes dalzieli*, *Aedes ochraceus*, and *Aedes vexans* serve as vectors in Senegal, and *Culex pipiens* in Egypt. Transovarial transmission has been found in *Aedes*, and epidemics may occur when high rainfall favors hatching and development of transovarially-infected offspring.

Clinical presentation: Disease is heralded by a flu-like illness with sudden onset of fever, headache, myalgia, and back pain. Nuchal rigidity and photophobia may also be present at this time. Complications include hemorrhagic fever on the second to fourth day of illness, or retinal hemorrhage or meningoencephalitis appearing after the first week. Hemorrhagic manifestations and fatal encephalitis have been observed in approximately 1 to 2% of patients during epidemics and account for much of the mortality. Retinitis occurs in 15% of patients. The case-fatality rate is 0.1%.

Specimens for diagnostic testing: blood, CSF, serum

Patient isolation precautions: blood precautions

Suggested assays for virus detection: detection of viral RNA by RT-PCR, virus isolation in cell cultures

Serodiagnosis: enzyme-linked immunosorbent assay for IgM and IgG antibodies, neutralization tests for confirmation

Biosafety level required for working with Rift Valley fever virus: BSL-3

Additional reading

Anon. An outbreak of Rift Valley Fever, eastern Africa, 1997–1998. Wkly Epidemiol Rec 1998;73:105–9.

Anon. Rift Valley Fever — East Africa, 1997–1998. MMWR Morb Mortal Wkly Rep 1998;47:261–4.

Anon. Rift Valley fever — Egypt, 1993. MMWR Morb Mort Wkly Rep 1994;43:693, 699–700.

Arthur RR, el Sharkawy MS, Cope SE, et al. Recurrence of Rift Valley fever in Egypt. Lancet 1993;342:1149–50.

Fontenille D, Traore Lamizana M, Diallo M, et al. New vectors of Rift Valley fever in West Africa. Emerg Infect Dis 1998;4:289–93.

http://www.who.int/emc/diseases/ebola/index.html (accessed September 21, 2002).

http://www.cdc.gov/ncidod/diseases/list_mosquitoborne.htm (accessed September 21, 2002).

http://www.emedicine.com/emerg/topic887.htm (accessed September 21, 2002).

Rocio encephalitis

Agent: Rocio virus, family Flaviviridae, genus *Flavivirus* (RNA)

Reservoir: possibly wild bird

Vector: mosquito (*Psorophora ferox*, *Aedes scapularis*)

Vehicle: none

Incubation period: average 12 d (range 7 d–15 d)

Clinical hints:

abdominal distention	neurological symptoms
conjunctivitis	pharyngitis
headache	vomiting

Typical therapy: symptomatic

Disease distribution: Brazil

Notes

Rocio virus was first described during an outbreak (465 cases, 6 fatal) in southern Sao Paulo State, Brazil, in 1975. The epidemic extended southward in 1976, resulting in an additional 825 cases and 95 deaths.

Human disease appears to be limited to Brazil. Most patients are males working in rural areas, with highest rates of infection occurring during March to May. Infection is most severe in young children and elderly adults.

Clinical presentation: A prodrome of fever, headache, malaise, vomiting, and conjunctivitis is followed by altered consciousness, motor weakness, and cerebellar dysfunction. One-third of patients progress to coma, and 10% die of the disease. Sequelae remain in 20% of survivors.

Specimens for diagnostic testing: brain tissue, serum

Patient isolation precautions: avoid access by mosquitoes

Suggested assays for virus detection: detection of viral RNA by RT-PCR, virus isolation in cell cultures

Serodiagnosis: enzyme-linked immunosorbent assays for IgM and IgG antibodies, neutralization tests for confirmation

Biosafety level required for working with Rocio virus: BSL-3

Additional reading

Burke DS, Monath TP. Flaviviruses. In: Knipe DM, Howley PM, editors. Fields virology. Vol 1. 4th ed. Philadelphia: Lippincott Williams & Wilkins; 2001. p. 1043–126.

de Souza Lopes O, Coimbra TL, de Abreu Sacchetta L, Calisher CH. Emergence of a new arbovirus disease in Brazil. I. Isolation and characterization of the etiologic agent, Rocio virus. Am J Epidemiol 1978;107:444–9.

de Souza Lopes O, de Abreu Sacchetta L, Francy DB, et al. Emergence of a new arbovirus disease in Brazil. III. Isolation of Rocio virus from *Psorophora ferox* (Humboldt, 1819). Am J Epidemiol 1981;113:122–5.

Lindenbach BD, Rice CM. Flaviviridae: the viruses and their replication. In: Knipe DM, Howley PM, editors. Fields virology. Vol 1. 4th ed. Philadelphia: Lippincott Williams & Wilkins; 2001. p. 991–1041.

Ross River disease

Agent: Ross River virus, family Togaviridae, genus *Alphavirus* (RNA)

Reservoirs: marsupials, horses, birds

Vector: mosquito (*Aedes vigilax*, *Culex annulirostris* also implicated)

Vehicle: none

Incubation period: 8 d–10 d (range 3 d–21 d)

Clinical hints:

arthralgia	maculopapular rash
headache	myalgia

Typical therapy: symptomatic

Disease distribution:

American Samoa	New Caledonia
Australia (Figure 7)	Papua New Guinea
Cook Islands	Samoa
Fiji	Solomon Islands
French Polynesia	Tonga
Indonesia	Wallis and Futuna Islands

Notes

Ross River disease has been found in Australia, Papua New Guinea, Indonesia, and the Pacific (Fiji, American Samoa, Cook Islands, New Caledonia).

An epidemic of approximately 50,000 cases involved several Pacific islands during 1979 to 1980, notably the Cook Islands, Fiji, New Caledonia, Samoa, and Wallis and Futuna.

Ross River disease 163

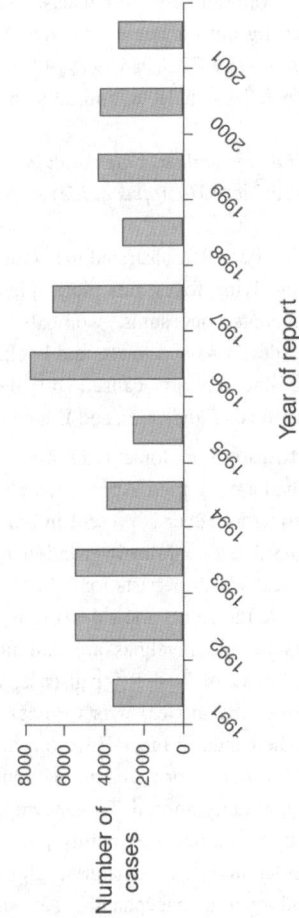

Figure 7 Ross River disease in Australia.

This is the most common arboviral disease in Australia, with most cases occurring during January to May. Yearly rates per 100,000 population were 22.9 in 1994, 14.9 in 1995, 42.9 in 1996, 35.9 in 1997, 16.7 in 1998, and 23.9 in 1999 and 21.9 in 2000.

Vectors include *Aedes vigilax*, *Culex annulirostris*, and *Aedes polynesiensis*. Wallabies (*Macropus agilis*) are suspected to act as reservoirs.

Seropositivity has been demonstrated in a wide variety of vertebrates, including flying foxes, rats, dogs, pigs, goats, sheep, kangaroos, bandicoots, opossums, wombats, potoroos, bettongs, Tasmanian devils, koalas, owls, and kookaburras.

Similar local illnesses are caused by **Barmah Forest** (*Alphavirus*), **Stratford** (*Flavivirus*), and **Edge Hill** (*Flavivirus*).

Clinical presentation: Symptomatic disease is more common among women than among men. Approximately 60% of infections are asymptomatic. Fever is present in only 30 to 50% of cases, and 50% develop a nonpruritic maculopapular rash of the trunk or extremities, which persists for 7 to 10 days. The rash occasionally involve the palms and soles, digits, face, and even the scalp. Headache and myalgias are common. Symmetric arthritis is the hallmark of Ross River disease, and tends to be severe and involves the ankles, wrists, knees, and interphalangeal joints of the hands and feet. Effusions are common and pain may persist for months or years, but without sequelae. The leukocyte count is usually normal. Tender lymphadenopathy is occasionally seen, as are lower extremity purpura, a vesicular rash, pruritis, splenomegaly, hematuria, glomerulonephritis, photophobia, and meningoencephalitis. No fatal cases have been reported.

Specimens for diagnostic testing: serum

Patient isolation precautions: avoid access by mosquitoes

Suggested assays for virus detection: detection of viral RNA by RT-PCR, virus isolation in cell cultures

Serodiagnosis: enzyme-linked immunosorbent assay for IgM and IgG antibodies, neutralization tests for confirmation

Biosafety level required for working with Ross River virus: BSL-2

Additional reading

Flexman JP, Smith DW, Mackenzie JS, et al. A comparison of the diseases caused by Ross River virus and Barmah Forest virus. Med J Aust 1998;169:159-63.

Griffin DE. Alphaviruses. In: Knipe DM, Howley PM, editors. Fields virology. Vol 1. 4th ed. Philadelphia: Lippincott Williams & Wilkins; 2001. p. 917–62.

Mackenzie JS, Broom AK, Hall RA, et al. Arboviruses in the Australian region, 1990 to 1998. Commun Dis Intell 1998;22:93–100.

Mackenzie JS, Smith DW. Mosquito-borne viruses and epidemic polyarthritis. Med J Aust 1996;164:90–3.

Sammels LM, Coelen RJ, Lindsay MD, Mackenzie JS. Geographic distribution and evolution of Ross River virus in Australia and the Pacific Islands. Virology 1995;212:20–9.

Schlesinger S, Schlesinger MJ. Togaviridae: the viruses and their replication. In: Knipe DM, Howley PM, editors. Fields virology. Vol 1. 4th ed. Philadelphia: Lippincott Williams & Wilkins; 2001. p. 895–916.

http://www.arbovirus.health.nsw.gov.au/arbovirus/viruses/rossriverbarmahforest.htm (accessed September 21, 2002).

http://medicineau.net.au/clinical/medicine/medicine3.html (accessed September 21, 2002).

Sindbis fever

Agent: Sindbis virus, family Togaviridae, genus *Alphavirus* (RNA)

Reservoir: wild birds

Vector: mosquito (*Culex univittatus* and *Culex tritaeniorhyncus*)

Vehicle: none

Incubation period: 3 d–6 d

Clinical hints:

arthritis
fever

myalgia
papular-to-vesicular rash

Typical therapy: symptomatic

Disease distribution:

Australia
Brunei
Czechoslovakia (former)
Egypt
India
Indonesia
Iran
Israel
Malaysia
Philippines
Russia (former Soviet Union)
Saudi Arabia
South Africa
Sri Lanka
Sudan
Thailand
Uganda

Similar diseases due to the same or essentially identical virus: **Karelian fever** in the former Soviet Union, **Ockelbo disease** in Sweden, and **Pogosta disease** in Finland (Figure 8).

Notes

Sindbis virus was first isolated from mosquitoes (*Culex univittatus*) in Egypt, in 1952. Human infections have been described

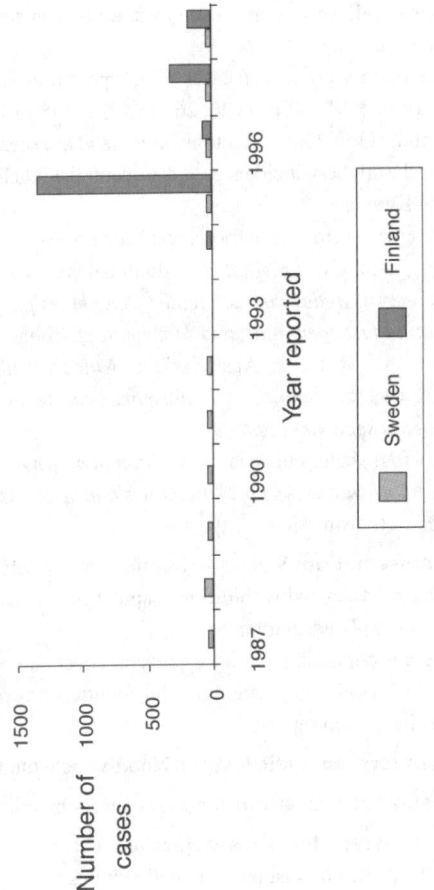

Figure 8 Sindbis fever in Sweden ("Ockelbo disease") and Finland ("Pagosta disease").

in Europe, Asia, Africa, and Australia. The virus has been isolated from a wide variety of mosquitoes, birds, hamsters, bats, frogs, mites, and ticks.

Three laboratory-confirmed cases were reported in Finland in 1994, 1,310 in 1995, 40 in 1996, 264 in 1997, 135 in 1998, 27 in 1999, and 123 in 2000. Infections in Finland are seen nationwide, but the highest incidences are in central Finland, Savo, and North Karelia.

The principal vectors in Africa are *Culex antennatus*, *Culex perexiguus*, and *Cx. univittatus*. Additional vectors include *Aedes cumminsi*, *Aedes circumluteolus*, *Anopheles pharoensis*, *Coquillettidia fuscopennatus*, and *Mansonia africana*.

The principal vector in Australasia is *Culex annulirostris*. Additional vectors include *Aedes normanensis*, *Aedes vigilax*, and *Mansonia septempuntata*.

The principal vectors in Asia are *Culex bitaeniorhynchus* and *Cx. tritaeniorhynchus*. *Culex pseudovishnui* has also been implicated in transmission.

Clinical presentation: Sindbis virus infection is a self-limited febrile illness associated with diffuse papular or vesicular rash, typically in the plantar region.

Arthralgia is common and may be severe. Fever and rash persist for 2 to 3 weeks and arthralgias for months or even years. No deaths have been reported.

Specimens for diagnostic testing: blood, vesicle fluid, serum

Patient isolation precautions: prevent access by mosquitoes

Suggested assays for virus detection: detection of viral RNA by RT-PCR, virus isolation in cell cultures

Serodiagnosis: enzyme-linked immunosorbent assays for IgM and IgG antibodies, neutralization tests for confirmation

Biosafety level required for working with Sindbis virus:
BSL-2

Additional reading

Francy DB, Jaenson TG, Lundstrom JO, et al. Ecologic studies of mosquitoes and birds as hosts of Ockelbo virus in Sweden and isolation of Inkoo and Batai viruses from mosquitoes. Am J Trop Med Hyg 1989;41:355–63.

Griffin DE. Alphaviruses. In: Knipe DM, Howley PM, editors. Fields virology. Vol 1. 4th ed. Philadelphia: Lippincott Williams & Wilkins; 2001. p. 917–62.

Lundstrom JO, Vene S, Espmark A, et al. Geographical and temporal distribution of Ockelbo disease in Sweden. Epidemiol Infect 1991;106:567–74.

Lvov DK, Skvortsova TM, Berezina LK, et al. Isolation of Karelian fever agent from *Aedes communis* mosquitoes [letter]. Lancet 1984;2:399–400.

Niklasson B, Vene S. Vector-borne viral diseases in Sweden a short review. Arch Virol 1996;11 Suppl:49-55.

Schlesinger S, Schlesinger MJ. Togaviridae: the viruses and their replication. In: Knipe DM, Howley PM, editors. Fields virology. Vol 1. 4th ed. Philadelphia: Lippincott Williams & Wilkins; 2001. p. 895–916.

Turunen M, Kuusisto P, Uggeldahl PE, Toivanen A. Pogosta disease: clinical observations during an outbreak in the province of North Karelia, Finland. Br J Rheumatol 1998;37:1177–80.

Spondweni fever

Agent: Spondweni virus, family Flaviviridae, genus *Flavivirus* (RNA)

Reservoir: unknown

Vector: mosquito (*Aedes circumluteolus*, *Armigeres*, *Culex*, *Eretmapodites*, and *Mansonia* spp), tick for Koutango virus

Vector: none

Incubation period: not known

Clinical hints:

fever	myalgia
headache	pruritic maculopapular rash

Typical therapy: symptomatic

Disease distribution:

Angola	Papua New Guinea
Botswana	Senegal
Burkina Faso	South Africa
Cameroon	Uganda
Nigeria	

Notes

Spondweni is named for the Spondweni region of South Africa. The virus appears to be widespread in Africa.

Although the natural cycle is not known, the causative agent is found in mosquitoes (notably *Aedes circumluteolus*); livestock may be seropositive.

Zika virus is a related agent responsible for cases of fever, rash, and arthralgia in Indonesia, Malaysia, and Africa (west, east, and central). As many as 50% of some African populations have antibody to Zika virus. *Aedes* spp serve as vectors for this virus, and monkeys as reservoirs.

Usutu virus and **Banzi** virus are African mosquito-borne flaviviruses belonging to the Spondweni and Uganda-S complexes, respectively. Symptoms of both diseases include fever and rash. **Usutu** virus is transmitted by mosquitoes of the genus *Culex*. Usutu virus has recently been detected in birds in central Europe; further epidemiologic developments are likely.

Sepik virus is a mosquito-borne agent of nonspecific illness in Papua New Guinea.

Koutango virus has been implicated in cases of fever, rash, and arthralgia in West and Central Africa. The virus has been isolated from rodents, and shown to be transmitted by ticks.

Clinical presentation: Spondweni is mild and symptoms are limited to fever, myalgia, and a maculopapular rash. Neither death nor sequelae have been reported.

Specimens for diagnostic testing: blood, serum

Patient isolation precautions: prevent access by mosquitoes

Suggested assays for virus detection: virus isolation in cell cultures

Serodiagnosis: enzyme-linked immunosorbent assays for IgM and IgG antibodies, neutralization tests for confirmation

Biosafety level required for working with Spondweni virus: BSL-3

Additional reading

Burke DS, Monath TP. Flaviviruses. In: Knipe DM, Howley PM, editors. Fields virology. Vol 1. 4th ed. Philadelphia: Lippincott Williams & Wilkins; 2001. p. 1043–126.

Lindenbach BD, Rice CM. Flaviviridae: the viruses and their replication. In: Knipe DM, Howley PM, editors. Fields virology. Vol 1. 4th ed. Philadelphia: Lippincott Williams & Wilkins; 2001. p. 991–1041.

Wolfe MS, Calisher CH, McGuire K. Spondweni virus infection in a foreign resident of Upper Volta. Lancet 1982;2:1306–8.

St. Louis encephalitis

Agent: St. Louis encephalitis virus, family Flaviviridae, genus *Flavivirus* (RNA)

Reservoir: bird, mammal

Vector: mosquito (*Culex pipiens*, *Culex tarsalis*, *Culex nigripalpus*, *Culex restuans*, *Culex salinarius*, *Aedes* spp, *Sabethes* spp)

Vehicle: none

Incubation period: 4 d–21 d

Clinical hints:

encephalitis
headache
meningitis
myalgia
photophobia
sore throat
vomiting

Typical therapy: symptomatic

Disease distribution:

Argentina
Belize
Brazil
Canada
Colombia
Costa Rica
Ecuador
El Salvador
Guatemala
Guyana
Haiti
Honduras
Jamaica
Mexico
Netherlands Antilles
Panama
Suriname
Trinidad & Tobago
United States
Uruguay
Venezuela

Notes

St. Louis encephalitis is found in the Americas, including the Caribbean area and until the recent invasion by West Nile virus, was considered the most important mosquito-borne disease in the United States. The first cases were described in St. Louis, Missouri, in 1933, during which 1,095 cases were registered.

Most cases are encountered during late summer; four cases were reported nationwide in the United States in 1999 (all from Florida), 3 in 2000, and 3 in 2001.

Important vectors include *Cx. tarsalis* in the western United States, *Cx. nigripalpus* in Florida, and *Cx. pipiens quinquefasciatus* in the Ohio-Mississippi River basins. Additional vectors include *Aedes dorsalis/melanimon*, *Aedes scapularis*, *Aedes serratus*, *Anopheles crucians*, *Culex peus*, *Cx. restuans*, and *Cx. salinarius*.

Clinical presentation: Overt infection and fatal infection are both ten times more common among elderly patients than among children. Five to ten percent of patients will suffer from chronic neurological sequelae. The disease may initially present with constitutional symptoms, aseptic meningitis, and overt and even fatal encephalitis. Infection begins with malaise, fever, headache, respiratory symptoms, diarrhea, vomiting, and myalgias. Symptoms may progress after several days to lethargy, confusion, tremor, clumsiness, and ataxia. General motor weakness is the rule, rather than focal neurological signs; however, 25% of patients develop cranial nerve signs. Signs of meningeal irritation are more common among children. Tremor and cerebellar signs are common. Seizures are uncommon, and carry a poor prognosis. Pneumonia, thrombophlebitis, pulmonary embolism, stroke, gastrointestinal hemorrhage, and nosocomial infections may also occur. Most cases resolve within 5 to 10 days. The case-fatality rate is 8%, with 20% being above the age of 60.

The peripheral leukocyte count may be slightly elevated, and hyponatremia occurs in more than 33% of patients. The CSF pressure is elevated in 33% of cases and the CSF protein in 70%. Between five to several hundred leukocytes per mm^3 are found.

Modoc virus and **Rio Bravo** virus are other flaviviruses that have been implicated in cases of aseptic meningitis in the western United States and in Canada. Modoc virus occurs in rodents, and Rio Bravo virus in bats. Accidental laboratory infection by Rio Bravo virus has been reported.

Specimens for diagnostic testing: brain tissue, CSF, serum

Patient isolation precautions: prevent access by mosquitoes

Suggested assays for virus detection: detection of viral RNA by RT-PCR, virus isolation in cell cultures

Serodiagnosis: enzyme-linked immunosorbent assays for IgM and IgG antibodies, neutralization tests for confirmation

Biosafety level required for working with St. Louis encephalitis virus: BSL-2

Additional reading

Anon. Arboviral disease — United States, 1994. MMWR Morb Mort Wkly Rep 1995;44:641–4.

Burke DS, Monath TP. Flaviviruses. In: Knipe DM, Howley PM, editors. Fields virology. Vol 1. 4th ed. Philadelphia: Lippincott Williams & Wilkins; 2001. p. 1043–126.

Ho DD, Hirsch MS. Acute viral encephalitis. Med Clin North Am 1985;69:415–29.

Lindenbach BD, Rice CM. Flaviviridae: the viruses and their replication. In: Knipe DM, Howley PM, editors. Fields virology. Vol 1. 4th ed. Philadelphia: Lippincott Williams & Wilkins; 2001. p. 991–1041.

Monath TP, Tsai TF. St. Louis encephalitis: lessons from the last decade. Am J Trop Med Hyg 1987;37 Suppl 3:S40–59.

Tsai TF. Arboviral infections in the United States. Infect Dis Clin North Am 1991;5:73–102.

http://www.cdc.gov/ncidod/dvbid/arbor/index.htm (accessed September 21, 2002).

http://www.cdc.gov/ncidod/diseases/list_mosquitoborne.htm (accessed September 21, 2002).

Tanapox virus disease

Agent: tanapox virus, family Poxviridae, genus *Yatapoxvirus* (DNA)

Reservoir: monkey

Vector: none

Vehicle: contact with monkey

Incubation period: not known

Clinical hints:

contact with monkeys
exposure to rain forest
fever
headache
thick-walled papules or vesicles

Typical therapy: symptomatic

Disease distribution: Democratic Republic of Congo, Kenya

Notes

Tanapox infection was first described on the Lower Tana River in Kenya during 1957.

Mechanical transmission probably occurs from monkey (notably vervets = *Cercopithecus aethiops*) to humans via mosquitoes. Human-to human transmission has not been documented.

Clinical presentation: The onset of illness is heralded by abrupt fever, occasionally with severe headache and prostration. A small number of umbilicated vesicles develop and are reminiscent of smallpox lesions; however, pustules are not encountered. Lesions contain a cheesy material, and are usually found on the upper trunk face and trunk, but not the feet, legs, or hands. Neither residua nor fatal infection have been reported.

Specimens for diagnostic testing: skin biopsy or exudate

Patient isolation precautions: prevent contact with infected lesions and exudates

Suggested assays for virus detection: detection of viral nucleic acid by RT-PCR, virus isolation in cell cultures

Serodiagnosis: enzyme-linked immunosorbent assays for IgM and IgG antibodies, neutralization tests for confirmation

Biosafety level required for working with tanapox virus: BSL-3

Additional reading

Axford JS, Downie AW. Tanapox. A serological survey of the lower Tana River Valley. J Hyg (London) 1979;83:273–6.

Downie AW, Taylor-Robinson CH, Caunt AE, et al. Tanapox: a new disease caused by a pox virus. Br Med J 1971;1:363–8.

Esposito JJ, Fenner F. Poxviruses. In: Knipe DM, Howley PM, editors. Fields virology. Vol 2. 4th ed. Philadelphia: Lippincott Williams & Wilkins; 2001. p. 2885–921.

Jezek Z, Arita I, Szczeniowski M, et al. Human tanapox in Zaire: clinical and epidemiological observations on cases confirmed by laboratory studies. Bull World Health Organ 1985;63:1027–35.

Moss B. Poxviridae: the viruses and their replication. In: Knipe DM, Howley PM, editors. Fields virology. Vol 2. 4th ed. Philadelphia: Lippincott Williams & Wilkins; 2001. p. 2849–83.

http://research.ucsb.edu/connect/pro/disease.html#v4 (accessed September 21, 2002).

Thogoto virus disease

Agent: Thogoto virus, family Orthomyxoviridae, genus *Thogotovirus* (RNA)

Reservoir: sheep, bird

Vector: tick

Vehicle: none

Incubation period: 4 d–5 d

Clinical hints:

contact with livestock	lymphadenopathy
encephalitis	optic neuritis
hepatitis	tick bite

Typical therapy: symptomatic

Disease distribution:

northern and southern Africa	Nigeria
southern Europe	Uganda
Kenya	Iran

Notes

Thogoto virus is found in northern and southern Africa, Iran, and southern Europe; however, human disease is rare and sporadic.

The life cycle of the virus is uncertain, but appears to involve livestock, ticks, and migratory birds. A single isolate has been recovered from a banded mongoose (*Mongos mungo*) in Uganda.

Fatal human infections have been reported, as have "abortion storms" in sheep.

The tick-borne **Dhori** virus is related to Thogoto virus, and has been associated with meningoencephalitis. During the

1980s, 5 cases of accidental human infections with Dhori virus were reported in the former Soviet Union. Clinical features consisted of an "acute course with marked general toxicity and a febrile period of 2-4 days." Two of the 5 patients developed "subcortical symptoms and mild involvement of the pyramidal system or encephalopolyradiculoneuritis with paresthesia and sensitivity disorders."

Clinical presentation: Detailed data on the clinical features of Thogoto virus have not been published. Encephalitis, optic neuritis and hepatitis have been reported, in some cases with fatal outcome.

Specimens for diagnostic testing: blood (not frozen), CSF, brain tissue, serum

Patient isolation precautions: none

Suggested assays for virus detection: detection of viral RNA by RT-PCR, virus isolation in cell cultures

Serodiagnosis: enzyme-linked immunosorbent assays for IgM and IgG antibodies, neutralization tests for confirmation

Biosafety level required for working with Thogoto virus: BSL-3

Additional reading

Calisher CH, Karabatsos N, Filipe AR. Antigenic uniformity of topotype strains of Thogoto virus from Africa, Europe, and Asia. Am J Trop Med Hyg 1987;37:670–3.

Davies FG, Soi RK, Wariru BN. Abortion in sheep caused by Thogoto virus. Vet Rec 1984;115:654.

Haig DA, Woodall JP, Danskin D. Thogoto virus: a hitherto undescribed agent isolated from ticks in Kenya. J Gen Microbiol 1965;38:389–94.

Jones LD, Davies CR, Steel GM, Nuttall PA. Vector capacity of *Rhipicephalus appendiculatus* and *Amblyomma variegatum* for Thogoto and Dhori viruses. Med Vet Entomol 1997;3: 195–202.

Moore DL, Causey OR, Carey DE, et al. Arthropod-borne viral infections of man in Nigeria, 1964–1970. Ann Trop Med Parasitol 1975;69:49–64.

Woodall J. Thogoto virus. In: Service MW, editor. Encyclopedia of arthropod-transmitted infections of man and domesticated animals. CAB International; 2001. p. 504–6.

Tick-borne encephalitis (Central European)
(European tick-borne encephalitis, Hanzalova virus disease, Hypr virus disease, Kumlinge virus disease, Neudoerfl virus disease)

Agent: Central European encephalitis virus, family Flaviviridae, genus *Flavivirus* (RNA)

Reservoir: ticks, rodents of many species, birds, cattle

Vector: tick (*Ixodes ricinus*)

Vehicle: dairy products

Incubation period: 7 d–14 d (range 4 d–20 d)

Clinical hints:

biphasic illness	myalgia
encephalitis	tick bite
headache	

Typical therapy: symptomatic

Disease distribution:

Austria	Italy
Bulgaria	Norway
Czechoslovakia (former)	Poland
Denmark	Romania
Finland	Russia (former Soviet Union)
France	Sweden
Germany	Switzerland
Greece	Turkey
Hungary	Yugoslavia (former)
Iran	

Notes

The viruses that cause European tick-borne encephalitis and Far Eastern tick-borne encephalitis are virtually identical; however, the two conditions have different geographic distributions, clinical presentations, and tick vectors. The European form (Central European encephalitis) is found in almost all the European countries.

Hundreds to thousands of cases occur annually. The disease is most common in forests, on hills or mountains. Cases occur during April to October, with highest rates during June to July. The average incidence in Europe is 1:100,000 per year. Outbreaks due to virus in goat and cow milk have been reported from Poland, Germany, the former Czechoslovakia, and Byelorussia.

Clinical presentation: Disease caused by Central European encephalitis virus is milder than that caused by Russian spring-summer encephalitis virus (Far Eastern encephalitis). Only 0.4% of infections are symptomatic, and only 5 to 30% of these will develop neurological disease. Illness begins with fever, malaise, headache, myalgia, and vomiting. These symptoms resolve spontaneously within 7 days. In cases of neurological disease, an asymptomatic interval of 1 to 20 days is followed by high fever, headache, and vomiting. In some cases, only aseptic meningitis or radiculitis follows; in others, the patient may have overt encephalitis, which is characterized by altered consciousness, ataxia, tremors, paresthesias, and focal signs. Seizures are relatively uncommon. Radiculitis tends to involve the shoulder girdle and upper limbs; however, bladder function and other autonomic functions can be disturbed. Bulbar involvement (cranial nerves III, VII, IX, X, and XI) results in paralysis of gaze and peripheral facial function, dysphagia, and dysarthria. Symptoms may persist for weeks following the acute infection.

The prognosis is generally favorable, especially among children. Sequelae are reported in up to 40% of patients, manifested as psychological and neurological disturbances such as asthenia, headache, memory loss, altered concentration, anxiety, emotional lability, ataxia, incoordination, tremor, and dysphasia. Residual cranial or spinal muscular paralysis persists in less than 5% of these patients. The case-fatality rate is less than 2%.

Specimens for diagnostic testing: brain tissue, CSF, blood (not frozen), serum

Patient isolation precautions: none

Suggested assays for virus detection: detection of viral RNA by RT-PCR, virus isolation in cell cultures

Serodiagnosis: enzyme-linked immunosorbent assays for IgM and IgG antibodies, neutralization tests for confirmation

Biosafety level required for working with Central European encephalitis virus: BSL-4

Additional reading

Anon. Tick-borne encephalitis and haemorrhagic fever with renal syndrome in Europe. Report on a WHO meeting. EURO Rep Stud 1986;1–79.

Anon. Tick-borne encephalitis. Wkly Epidemiol Rec 1995;70:120–2.

Burke DS, Monath TP. Flaviviruses. In: Knipe DM, Howley PM, editors. Fields virology. Vol 1. 4th ed. Philadelphia: Lippincott Williams & Wilkins; 2001. p. 1043–126.

Calisher CH. Antigenic classification and taxonomy of flaviviruses (family Flaviviridae) emphasizing a universal system for the taxonomy of viruses causing tick-borne encephalitis. Acta Virol 1988;32:469–78.

Dumpis U, Crook D, Oksi J. Tick-borne encephalitis. Clin Infect Dis 1999;28:882–90.

Kunz C. Tick-borne encephalitis in Europe. Acta Leiden 1992;60:1–14.

Lindenbach BD, Rice CM. Flaviviridae: the viruses and their replication. In: Knipe DM, Howley PM, editors. Fields virology. Vol 1. 4th ed. Philadelphia: Lippincott Williams & Wilkins; 2001. p. 991-1041.

http://www.cdc.gov/ncidod/dvbid/arbor/index.htm (accessed September 21, 2002).

Tick-borne encephalitis (Russian spring-summer)
(Far Eastern tick-borne encephalitis)

Agent: Russian spring-summer encephalitis virus, family Flaviviridae, genus *Flavivirus* (RNA)

Reservoir: rodents, ticks, goats, cattle

Vector: tick (*Ixodes persulcatus*)

Vehicle: dairy products

Incubation period: 7 d–14 d (range 4 d–20 d)

Clinical hints:

encephalitis	headache
follows tick bite	myalgia

Typical therapy: symptomatic

Disease distribution:

Bulgaria	Japan
China	Korea
Iran	Russia (eastern former Soviet Union)

Notes

Far Eastern tick-borne encephalitis was first described during the 1930s in the former Soviet Union. Rates peak during May to June, and August to September. Occupational contact accounts for 15 to 20% of cases, and urban residents for 70%. Unboiled goat milk is no longer an important source for infection.

The viruses that cause European tick-borne encephalitis and Far Eastern tick-borne encephalitis are nearly identical, but have epidemiologic and clinical differences.

Negishi virus was first isolated in 1948 from a child with encephalitis in Japan. Natural foci of infection are found on

Hokkaido, Japan, and seropositive populations have been demonstrated in the Khabarovsk region of Russia.

A related virus, **Tyuleniy** virus, is thought to infect humans, and is found among sea birds and ticks (*Ixodes putus* and *Ixodes uriae*) on Tyuleniy Island (Sea of Okhotsk), the Barentsev coastline of Kolsky Peninsula, Norway, and the United States.

Meaban virus has been implicated in a case of lymphadenopathy associated with arthralgia, purpura, and tonsillitis. Meaban virus is found in France and Russia.

Alma-Arasan is a flavivirus infection characterized by fever and meningitis. Cases have been described in Kazakhstan. The local vector is thought to be *Ixodes persulcatus*.

Yet another flavivirus, **Karshi** virus, has been reported to cause a nonspecific febrile illness in Uzbekistan. The agent is transmitted by various tick species, and has a reservoir in rodents.

Clinical presentation: Far Eastern tick-borne encephalitis is more severe than the Central European variety, and is associated with case-fatality rates of 20% among hospitalized cases, and neurologic sequelae in up to 60%. Unlike the Central European form, the illness is monophasic, presenting with hectic fever, severe headache, vomiting, photophobia, nuchal rigidity, stupor, focal neurological deficits, seizures, and coma. Involvement of the brain stem grey matter and upper spinal cord produces cranial nerve palsies, respiratory and cardiac disturbances, brachial plexus, and neck weakness with residual atrophy. Sequelae include progressive motor weakness and intractable seizures.

Specimens for diagnostic testing: brain tissue, CSF, blood (not frozen), serum

Patient isolation precautions: none

Suggested assays for virus detection: detection of viral RNA by RT-PCR, virus isolation in cell cultures

Serodiagnosis: enzyme-linked immunosorbent assays for IgM and IgG antibodies, neutralization tests for confirmation

Biosafety level required for working with Russian spring-summer encephalitis virus: BSL-4

Additional reading

Anon. Tick-borne encephalitis and haemorrhagic fever with renal syndrome in Europe. Report on a WHO meeting. EURO Rep Stud 1986;1–79.

Anon. Tick-borne encephalitis. Wkly Epidemiol Rec 1995;70: 120–2.

Calisher CH. Antigenic classification and taxonomy of flaviviruses (family Flaviviridae) emphasizing a universal system for the taxonomy of viruses causing tick-borne encephalitis. Acta Virol 1988;32:469–78.

Dumpis U, Crook D, Oksi J. Tick-borne encephalitis. Clin Infect Dis 1999;28:882–90.

Kunz C. Tick-borne encephalitis in Europe. Acta Leiden 1992; 60:1–14.

http://www.cdc.gov.nciod/dvbid/arbor/index.htm (accessed September 21, 2002).

Venezuelan equine encephalitis (VEE)
(Peste loca)

Agent: Venezuelan equine encephalitis virus, family Togaviridae, genus *Alphavirus* (RNA)

Reservoir: rodent, horse

Vector: mosquito (*Culex* [*Melanoconion*] spp, *Aedes taeniorhynchus*, *Psorophora confinnis*, others during epizootics)

Vehicle: none

Incubation period: 2 d–5 d (range 1 d–6 d)

Clinical hints:

arthralgia	fever
conjunctivitis	myalgia
encephalitis	vomiting

Typical therapy: symptomatic

Disease distribution:

Argentina	Honduras
Bolivia	Mexico
Brazil	Netherlands Antilles
Colombia	Panama
Costa Rica	Peru
Ecuador	Suriname
El Salvador	Trinidad & Tobago
French Guiana	United States
Guatemala	Venezuela
Guyana	

Considered a potential bioterrorism weapon.

Notes

The virus of Venezuelan equine encephalitis was first isolated in Venezuela, Aragua State, in 1938, and has been responsible for epizootics and epidemics in 12 countries in the area as of 1996. Five subtype I viruses are recognized; at least three of them (VEE IA-B, ID and IE) are pathogenic for humans. Incompletely inactivated vaccines have been implicated in some outbreaks.

Everglades virus (VEE II) has been shown to cause a few human illnesses.

Tonate virus (VEE type IIIB) has been reported to cause an undifferentiated febrile illness. A single fatal case of Tonate virus infection was reported in French Guiana.

Eleven epidemics were reported between 1935 and 1961, and yearly epidemics were reported during 1962 to 1973. The largest epidemic of VEE IA-B virus was described beginning in 1969, and affected Ecuador, Venezuela, Central America, Mexico, and, by 1971, Texas. The last cases were reported in Mexico in 1972.

Other mosquito species from which these viruses have been isolated include *Aedes serratus*, *Ae. taeniorhynchus*, and more than 35 other species of *Aedes*, *Anopheles*, *Culex*, *Deinoceritis*, *Haemagogus*, *Limatus*, *Mansonia*, *Psorophora*, *Sabethes*, and *Wyeomyia*.

Clinical presentation: See Eastern equine encephalitis. VEE is often characterized by a mild flu-like illness in endemic countries, and 40% of patients are asymptomatic. Overt infection is heralded by fever, chills, myalgia, headache with or without photophobia, hyperesthesia, and vomiting. Sore throat is noted in some cases. Four percent of children and less than 1% of adults progress to overt encephalitis, a few days to a week following the prodrome. Encephalitis is characterized by nuchal rigidity, ataxia, convulsions, coma, and paralysis. Lymphopenia is common, often associated with neutropenia and mild thrombocytopenia. Hepatic dysfunction is common, and CSF examination reveals a few hundred lymphocytes. The case-fatality rate is less than 1%, but increases to 20% in cases of encephalitis.

Specimens for diagnostic testing: brain tissue, CSF, serum

Patient isolation precautions: avoid access by mosquitoes

Suggested assays for virus detection: detection of viral RNA by RT-PCR, virus isolation in cell cultures

Serodiagnosis: enzyme-linked immunosorbent assays for IgM and IgG antibodies, neutralization tests for confirmation

Biosafety level required for working with Venezuelan equine encephalitis viruses: BSL-3

Additional reading

Anon. Update: Venezuelan equine encephalitis — Colombia, 1995. MMWR Morb Mort Wkly Rep 1995;44:775–7.

Griffin DE. Alphaviruses. In: Knipe DM, Howley PM, editors. Fields virology. Vol 1. 4th ed. Philadelphia: Lippincott Williams & Wilkins; 2001. p. 917–62.

Hommel D, Heraud JM, Hulin A, Talarmin A. Association of Tonate virus (subtype IIIB of the Venezuelan equine encephalitis complex) with encephalitis in a human. Clin Infect Dis 2000;30:188–90.

Rico-Hesse R, Weaver SC, de Siger J, et al. Emergence of a new epidemic/epizootic Venezuelan equine encephalitis virus in South America. Proc Natl Acad Sci U S A 1995;92:5278–81.

Rivas F, Diaz LA, Cardenas VM, et al. Epidemic Venezuelan equine encephalitis in La Guajira, Colombia, 1995. J Infect Dis 1997;175:828–32.

Schlesinger S, Schlesinger MJ. Togaviridae: the viruses and their replication. In: Knipe DM, Howley PM, editors. Fields virology. Vol 1. 4th ed. Philadelphia: Lippincott Williams & Wilkins; 2001. p. 895–916.

Weaver SC, Salas R, Rico Hesse R, et al. Re-emergence of epidemic Venezuelan equine encephalomyelitis in South America. Lancet 1996;348:436–40.

http://www.emedicine.com/emerg/topic886.htm (accessed September 21, 2002).

Venezuelan hemorrhagic fever

Agent: Guanarito virus, family Arenaviridae, genus *Arenavirus* (RNA), Tacaribe complex

Reservoir: cane mouse (*Zygodontomys brevicauda*), possibly other rodents (cotton rat: *Sigmodon alstoni*)

Vector: none

Vehicle: possibly excreta

Incubation period: not known

Clinical hints:

arthralgia	leukopenia
headache	pharyngitis
hemorrhagic diathesis	thrombocytopenia

Typical therapy: symptomatic

Disease distribution: Venezuela

Considered a potential bioterrorism weapon.

Notes

Venezuelan hemorrhagic fever (VHF) was first reported as an outbreak (15 cases, 9 fatal) in Portuguesa State during 1989. Subsequent cases were reported from Barinas State. To date, this disease has been limited to Venezuela.

Highest rates (41% of cases) are reported during December to January.

The clinical features of VHF are similar to those of Argentine hemorrhagic fever (q.v.); however, pharyngitis is common in VHF.

The local reservoir appears to be the cane mouse (*Z. brevicauda*). Cotton rats (*S.alstoni*) are infected by a related *Arenavirus* (**Pirital** virus) of unknown significance to humans.

Clinical presentation: The onset of the illness is gradual, and characterized by fever, pharyngitis, and myalgia. Additional findings include abdominal pain, headache, dizziness, photophobia, and constipation. Conjunctivitis and erythema of the face and trunk may appear. Petechiae and generalized lymphadenopathy are common. Hemorrhagic diatheses and neurological symptoms may appear, and the patient may exhibit mucosal bleeding, shock, pulmonary infiltration and edema, ataxia, tremors, seizures, and coma. The case-fatality rate is 30 to 40%.

Specimens for diagnostic testing: serum, liver, spleen

Patient isolation precautions: strict isolation

Suggested assays for virus detection: detection of viral RNA by RT-PCR, virus isolation in cell cultures

Serodiagnosis: enzyme-linked immunosorbent assays for IgM and IgG antibodies

Biosafety level required for working with Guanarito virus: BSL-4

Additional reading

Buchmeier MJ, Bowen MD, Peters CJ. Arenaviridae: the viruses and their replication. In: Knipe DM, Howley PM, editors. Fields virology. Vol 2. 4th ed. Philadelphia: Lippincott Williams & Wilkins; 2001. p. 1635–68.

de Manzione N, Salas RA, Paredes H, et al. Venezuelan hemorrhagic fever: clinical and epidemiological studies of 165 cases. Clin Infect Dis 1988;26:308–13.

Tesh RB. The emerging epidemiology of Venezuelan hemorrhagic fever and Oropouche fever in tropical South America. Ann N Y Acad Sci 1994;740:129–37.

Tesh RB, Wilson ML, Salas R, et al. Field studies on the epidemiology of Venezuelan hemorrhagic fever: implication of the cotton rat *Sigmodon alstoni* as the probable rodent reservoir. Am J Trop Med Hyg 1993;49:227–35.

Vainrub B, Salas R. Latin American hemorrhagic fever. Infect Dis Clin North Am 1994;8:47–59.

http://www.cdc.gov/ncidod/dvrd/spb/mnpages/dispages/arena.htm (accessed September 21, 2002).

http://www.emedicine.com/emerg/topic887.htm (accessed September 21, 2002).

Vesicular stomatitis

Agent: any of a number of related viruses, family Rhabdoviridae, genus *Vesiculovirus* (RNA)

Reservoir: horse, cattle, pig

Vector: flies and gnats (*Lutzomyia* spp and *Simulium* spp) may act as mechanical vectors

Vehicle: aerosol from animal

Incubation period: 2 d–6 d (range 1 d–8 d)

Clinical hints:

animal contact	myalgia
conjunctivitis	oral and digital vesicles
headache	

Typical therapy: symptomatic

Disease distribution:

Brazil	Panama
Canada	Senegal
India	United States
Mexico	

Notes

Vesicular stomatitis is a disease of domestic livestock. These include: cattle, which may develop secondary bacterial mastitis; swine, similar to swine vesicular disease and vesicular exanthema; and horses, which may develop lameness.

Human disease is not uncommon among animal handlers and laboratory personnel. Seropositivity is also found among rural populations, such as tropical America and Central Asia, even in the absence of known animal contact.

Viral serotypes include **Chandipura** (India), **Piry** (Brazil), **vesicular stomatitis Indiana**, **vesicular stomatitis New Jersey** (United States, Mexico, Central, and South America), and **vesicular stomatitis Alagoas** and **Cocal** (South America). The cattle disease is clinically indistinguishable from foot-and-mouth disease, and this differentiation must be made as quickly as possible.

Clinical presentation: Human disease is often mild, transitory, and nonspecific; however, at least two cases of severe encephalitis (Chandipura and vesicular stomatitis Indiana viruses) have been reported. In some cases, a biphasic illness is observed. Prominent findings include headache, myalgias, pharyngitis in 40% of cases, conjunctivitis, and cervical lymphadenopathy. Vesicles or ulcers are found in a minority of patients, appearing on the oral mucosa, lips, tongue, fingers, or nose. The infection resolves within 1 week. Neither fatal infection nor residua have been reported.

Specimens for diagnostic testing: blood, serum

Patient isolation precautions: none

Suggested assays for virus detection: detection of viral RNA by RT-PCR, virus isolation in cell cultures

Serodiagnosis: enzyme-linked immunosorbent assays for IgM and IgG antibodies, neutralization tests for confirmation

Biosafety level required for working with vesicular stomatitis viruses (except vesicular stomatitis Alagoas and Cocal viruses): BSL-3

Additional reading

de Mattos CA, de Mattos CC, Rupprecht CE. Rhabdoviruses. In: Knipe DM, Howley PM, editors. Fields virology. Vol 1. 4th ed. Philadelphia: Lippincott Williams & Wilkins; 2001. p. 1245–77.

Fields BN, Hawkins K. Human infection with the virus of vesicular stomatitis during an epizootic. N Engl J Med 1967; 277:989–94.

Hanson RP, Rasmussen AF, Brandley CA, Brown JW. Human infection with the virus of vesicular stomatitis. J Lab Clin Med 1950;36:754–8.

Reif JS, Webb PA, Monath TP, et al. Epizootic vesicular stomatitis in Colorado, 1982: infection in occupational risk groups. Am J Trop Med Hyg 1987;36:177–82.

Tesh RB, Peralta PH, Johnson KM. Ecologic studies of vesicular stomatitis virus. I. Prevalence of infection among animals and humans living in an area of endemic VSV activity. Am J Epidemiol 1969;90:255–61.

http://www.oie.int/eng/maladies/fiches/A_A020.htm (accessed September 21, 2002).

Wesselsbron disease

Agent: Wesselsbron virus, family Flaviridae, genus *Flavivirus* (RNA)

Reservoir: sheep, cattle

Vector: mosquito (*Aedes* spp, *Anopheles gambiae*, *Anopheles pharoensis*, *Culex telesilla*, *Culex univittatus*, *Mansonia uniformis*)

Vehicle: none

Incubation period: 2 d–4 d

Clinical hints:

arthralgia	leukopenia
dermal hyperesthesia	maculopapular rash
fever	myalgia

Typical therapy: symptomatic

Disease distribution:

Angola	Kenya
Botswana	Liberia
Cameroon	Madagascar
Chad	Malawi
Congo	Mozambique
Democratic Republic of Congo	Namibia
	Niger
Ethiopia	Nigeria
Gabon	Rwanda
Gambia	Senegal
Ghana	Sierra Leone
Guinea	Somalia
Ivory Coast	South Africa

Tanzania
Togo
Uganda
Zambia
Zimbabwe

Notes

The virus that causes Wesselsbron disease is widely distributed in sub-Saharan Africa, and is an important cause of disease in sheep.

Antibody to Wesselsbron is common among horses, camels, donkeys, and sheep, with lower rates among pigs and goats, notably in forest swamp zones.

Clinical presentation: Illness is characterized by abrupt onset of fever, myalgias, arthralgias, dermal hyperesthesia, leukopenia, and a maculopapular rash that appears 3 to 4 days after onset. Meningoencephalitis may follow. The disease lasts for up to 10 days. Although human infection may be severe, no fatalities have been reported.

Specimens for diagnostic testing: throat swabs, blood, serum

Patient isolation precautions: avoid access by mosquitoes

Suggested assays for virus detection: virus isolation in cell cultures

Serodiagnosis: enzyme-linked immunosorbent assays for IgM and IgG antibodies, neutralization tests for confirmation

Biosafety level required for working with Wesselsbron virus: BSL-3

Additional reading

Burke DS, Monath TP. Flaviviruses. In: Knipe DM, Howley PM, editors. Fields virology. Vol 1. 4th ed. Philadelphia: Lippincott Williams & Wilkins; 2001. p. 1043–126.

Fagbami A. Epidemiological investigations on arbovirus infections at Igbo-Ora, Nigeria. Trop Geogr Med 1977;29:187–91.

Guilherme JM, Gonella Legall C, Legall F, et al. Seroprevalence of five arboviruses in Zebu cattle in the Central African Republic. Trans R Soc Trop Med Hyg 1996;90:31–3.

Lindenbach BD, Rice CM. Flaviviridae: the viruses and their replication. In: Knipe DM, Howley PM, editors. Fields virology. Vol 1. 4th ed. Philadelphia: Lippincott Williams & Wilkins; 2001. p. 991–1041.

Rodhain F, Gonzalez JP, Mercier E, et al. Arbovirus infections and viral haemorrhagic fevers in Uganda: a serological survey in Karamoja district, 1984. Trans R Soc Trop Med Hyg 1989;83:851–4.

Tomori O, Monath TP, O'Connor EH, et al. Arbovirus infections among laboratory personnel in Ibadan, Nigeria. Am J Trop Med Hyg 1981;30:855–61.

West Nile virus fever, West Nile virus encephalitis
(Lourdige, Near Eastern equine encephalitis)

Agent: West Nile virus, family Flaviridae, genus *Flavivirus* (RNA)

Reservoir: birds, horses, bats, possibly ticks

Vector: mosquito (*Culex univittatus*, *Culex pipiens*, *Culex pipiens/restuans*, *Culex salinarius*, *Culex vishnui*, *Culex neavei*, *Coquillettidia spp*, *Ochlerotatus* [formerly *Aedes*] *japonicus*, *Ochlerotatus triseriatus*, *Ochlerotatus trivittatus*, *Aedes vexans*, *Aedes albopictus*, *Aedes* spp, *Culiseta melanura*, *Psorophora ferox*, and *Anopheles* spp; other species undoubtedly will be shown to be involved in the natural cycle of this virus in the United States)

Vehicle: none

Incubation period: 3 d–6 d (range 1 d–7 d)

Clinical hints:

arthralgia	macular rash
conjunctivitis	meningitis
encephalitis	muscle weakness
headache	myalgia
lymphadenopathy	myocarditis

Typical therapy: symptomatic

Disease distribution:

Albania	Canada
Algeria	Canary Islands
Austria	Cayman Islands
Botswana	Central African Republic
Bulgaria	China

Cyprus	Monaco
Czechoslovakia (former)	Morocco
Democratic Republic of Congo	Mozambique
	Namibia
Egypt	Nigeria
Ethiopia	Pakistan
France	Philippines
Gibraltar	Portugal
Greece	Romania
Hungary	Russia (former Soviet Union)
India	Senegal
Indonesia	South Africa
Iran	Spain
Iraq	Sri Lanka
Israel	Sudan
Italy	Syria
Ivory Coast	Thailand
Jordan	Tunisia
Kenya	Turkey
Lebanon	Uganda
Madagascar	United States
Malaysia	Yugoslavia (former)

Considered a potential bioterrorism weapon.

Notes

West Nile fever was first reported in the West Nile district of Uganda in 1937. West Nile virus (WNV) has a wider geographic distribution than any other flavivirus, with the exception of dengue viruses. Human disease is reported from much of Africa, the former Soviet Union, the Near East, India, Indonesia, and parts of Europe. In 1999 and 2000, outbreaks were reported in New York City and surrounding areas; the 1999 outbreak presumably was initiated by infected mosquitoes or humans. Twenty-one cases (2 fatal) were reported in 2000; 66 (9 fatal) in 2001; and over 2,400 (117 fatal) in 32 states during 2002. As of this writing, the virus has been detected in birds, mosquitoes and mammals in 43 states. It is expected that this virus will continue to spread throughout North America and possibly reach South America.

European disease occurs during July to September.

Although the principal reservoirs are wild birds, seropositive bats, camels, cattle, chimpanzees, chipmunks, dogs, fowl, horses, lemurs, monkeys, rabbits, raccoons, bears, goats, sheep, alpaca, wolves, squirrels, and skunks have also been identified. An enzootic cycle may persist among horses infected by moquitoes feeding on migrating white storks (*Ciconia ciconia*) in the Middle East.

The principal vector in Africa is *Culex univittatus*. Additional vectors include *Culex theileri*, *Culex weschei*, and *Coquillettidia metallica*.

The European vectors are *Culex modestus*, *Culex pipiens*, and *Coquillettidia richiardii*.

Vectors in the Middle East include *Anopheles coustani*, *Culex antennatus*, *Culex perexiguus*, and *Cx. pipiens* group.

The principal vector in the United States may be *Cx. pipiens*. Additional vectors include *Culex restuans* and *Culex salinarius* (dusk-to-dawn feeders). The virus is also found in *Ochlerotatus* (formerly *Aedes*) *japonicus*, *Ochlerotatus triseriatus* (daytime biters), *Ochlerotatus trivittatus*, *Aedes vexans*, *Aedes albopictus*, *Culiseta melanura*, *Psorophora ferox*, and *Anopheles punctipennis*. The natural history and life cycle of WNV in the New World is unclear at the time of this writing.

Viral RNA has also been detected in overwintering mosquitoes.

Asian vectors include *Anopheles subpictus*, *Culex quinquefasciatus*, *Culex tritaeniorhynchus*, and *Culex vishnui* group. The virus has also been isolated from ticks (*Argas hermanni* in Egypt and *Hyalomma* spp in the former Soviet Union).

Clinical presentation: West Nile fever in humans usually is a minor flu-like illness, characterized by an abrupt onset of moderate to high fever lasting 3 to 5 days. The fever is occasionally biphasic, and may be accompanied by rigors. Additional symptoms include frontal headache, sore throat, backache, myalgia, arthralgia, fatigue, conjunctivitis, and retrobulbar pain. A maculopapular or roseolar rash appears in approximately 50% of cases, spreading from the trunk to the extremities and head. Other symptoms include lymphadenopathy, anorexia, nausea, abdominal pain, diarrhea, and respiratory symptoms. Occasionally, in less than 15% of cases, acute aseptic meningitis or encephalitis occurs, associated with neck stiffness, vomiting, confusion, disturbed consciousness, somnolence, tremor of extremities, abnormal reflexes, convulsions, pareses, muscle weakness, and coma. Such patients may then develop anterior myelitis. Hepatosplenomegaly, hepatitis, pancreatitis, and myocarditis also occur. The milder form of the illness resolves within 1 week in most cases.

Laboratory findings consist of a slightly increased sedimentation rate and mild leukocytosis. Cerebrospinal fluid in patients with central nervous system involvement is clear, with moderate pleocytosis and elevated protein. The virus can be recovered from the blood for up to 10 days in immunocompetent febrile patients, and as late as 22 to 28 days after infection in immunocompromised patients. Peak viremia (never high) occurs 4 to 8 days postinfection. Recovery is complete, although less rapid in adults than in children, and often accompanied by long-term myalgias and weakness. Permanent sequelae have not been reported. Most fatal cases occur in patients older than 50 years.

Specimens for diagnostic testing: blood (not frozen), CSF, serum

Patient isolation precautions: none

Suggested assays for virus detection: detection of viral RNA by RT-PCR, virus isolation in cell cultures

Serodiagnosis: enzyme-linked immunosorbent assays for IgM and IgG antibodies, neutralization tests for confirmation

Biosafety level required for working with West Nile virus: BSL-3

Additional reading

Anon. Update: West Nile-like viral encephalitis — New York, 1999. Morb Mort Wkly Rep 1999;48:890–2.

Anon. Update: West Nile virus activity — Northeastern United States, January–August 7, 2000. MMWR Morb Mort Wkly Rep 2000;49:714–8.

Griffin DE. Alphaviruses. In: Knipe DM, Howley PM, editors. Fields virology. Vol 1. 4th ed. Philadelphia: Lippincott Williams & Wilkins; 2001. p. 917–62.

Hubalek Z, Halouzka J. West Nile fever — a reemerging mosquito-borne viral disease in Europe. Emerg Infect Dis 1999;5:643–50.

Lanciotti RS, Roehrig JT, Deubel V, et al. Origin of the West Nile virus responsible for an outbreak of encephalitis in the northeastern United States. Science 1999;286:2333–7.

Rappole JH, Derrickson SR, Hubalek Z. Migratory birds and spread of West Nile virus in the Western Hemisphere. Emerg Infect Dis 2000;6:319–28.

Savage HM, Ceianu C, Nicolescu G, et al. Entomologic and avian investigations of an epidemic of West Nile fever in Romania in 1996, with serologic and molecular characterization of a virus isolate from mosquitoes. Am J Trop Med Hyg 1999;61:600–11.

Schlesinger S, Schlesinger MJ. Togaviridae: the viruses and their replication. In: Knipe DM, Howley PM, editors. Fields virology. Vol 1. 4th ed. Philadelphia: Lippincott Williams & Wilkins; 2001. p. 895–916.

http://www.cdc.gov/ncidod/dvbid/arbor/index.htm (accessed September 21, 2002).

http://www.cdc.gov/ncidod/diseases/list_mosquitoborne.htm (accessed September 21, 2002).

http://www.cdc.gov/ncidod/dvbid/westnile/index.htm (accessed September 21, 2002).

Western equine encephalitis

Agent: western equine encephalitis virus, family Togaviridae, genus *Alphavirus* (RNA)

Reservoir: birds, possibly amphibians and reptiles

Vector: mosquito (*Culex tarsalis*)

Vehicle: none

Incubation period: 5 d–15 d

Clinical hints:

back pain	meningitis
encephalitis	vomiting
headache	

Typical therapy:

Disease distribution:

Argentina	Mexico
Brazil	United States
Canada	Uruguay
Guyana	

Considered a potential bioterrorism weapon.

Notes

Subtypes of western equine encephalitis virus occur throughout the western hemisphere. Clinical disease is relatively uncommon in South America, suggesting either lower transmission or lower pathogenic potential.

In temperate regions, the disease is most often encountered in late summer and autumn. and affects horses and humans.

Culex tarsalis, rarely found in the eastern United States, is responsible for enzootic transmission in western America.

Species of *Aedes*, *Anopheles*, *Culex*, *Culiseta*, and *Psorophora* are also implicated.

Clinical presentation: See eastern equine encephalitis. Case-to-infection ratios are approximately 1:1,000 for adults, 1:60 for children, and 1:1 for infants. Younger patients tend to suffer more severe disease, with rapid onset of symptoms, presence of seizures, and permanent neurological residua.

Specimens for diagnostic testing: serum, CSF, brain tissue

Patient isolation precautions: none

Suggested assays for virus detection: detection of viral RNA by RT-PCR, virus isolation in cell cultures

Serodiagnosis: enzyme-linked immunosorbent assays for IgM and IgG antibodies, neutralization tests for confirmation

Biosafety level required for working with western equine encephalitis virus: BSL-2

Additional reading

Anon. Arboviral disease — United States, 1994. MMWR Morb Mort Wkly Rep 1995;44:641–4.

Anon. Western equine encephalitis — United States and Canada, 1987. MMWR Morb Mort Wkly Rep 1987;36:655–9.

Calisher CH. Medically important arboviruses of the United States and Canada. Clin Microbiol Rev 1994;7:89–116.

Griffin DE. Alphaviruses. In: Knipe DM, Howley PM, editors. Fields virology. Vol 1. 4th ed. Philadelphia: Lippincott Williams & Wilkins; 2001. p. 917–62.

Reisen WK, Chiles RE. Prevalence of antibodies to western equine encephalomyelitis and St. Louis encephalitis viruses in residents of California exposed to sporadic and consistent enzootic transmission. Am J Trop Med Hyg 1997;57:526–9.

Schlesinger S, Schlesinger MJ. Togaviridae: the viruses and their replication. In: Knipe DM, Howley PM, editors. Fields virology. Vol 1. 4th ed. Philadelphia: Lippincott Williams & Wilkins; 2001. p. 895–916.

Tsai TF. Arboviral infections in the United States. Infect Dis Clin North Am 1991;5:73–102.

http://www.cdc.gov/ncidod/dvbid/arbor/index.htm (accessed September 21, 2002).

http://www.cdc.gov/ncidod/diseases/list_mosquitoborne.htm (accessed September 21, 2002).

Whitewater Arroyo virus infection

Agent: Whitewater Arroyo virus, family Arenaviridae, genus *Arenavirus* (RNA)

Reservoir: rodent (woodrats/packrats: *Neotoma* spp, particularly *albigula*)

Vector: none

Vehicle: possibly excreta

Incubation period: not known

Clinical hints:

acute respiratory distress syndrome (ARDS)	liver failure
	lymphopenia
fever	myalgia
headache	thrombocytopenia
hemorrhagic manifestations	

Typical therapy: symptomatic

Disease distribution: United States

Notes

During June 1999 to May 2000, two female patients in the United States were reported as having an illness caused by Whitewater Arroyo virus. One resided in southern California and the other in the San Francisco Bay area. No common source was found, and neither had traveled outside California during the 4 weeks preceding their illnesses. One had been in contact with rodent droppings. These cases have not been definitively confirmed as Whitewater Arroyo virus.

Viral RT-PCR analysis implicated an agent identical or similar to Whitewater Arroyo virus, an arenavirus that had been recovered from a white-throated woodrat (*Neotoma albigula*) from New Mexico during the early 1990s. Of 20 known species of *Neotoma*, 9 occur in the United States. The geographic range of these species incorporates most of the United States. At least five of the US species could potentially harbor the virus. In Colorado, 42.9% of female and 26.8% of male white-throated woodrats were seropositive between 1995 and 1999. Whitewater Arroyo virus has been detected in 3.3% of woodrats tested in the southwestern United States; seropositive rodents have been detected essentially throughout the western United States, but these may represent Whitewater Arroyo virus infections or infections with other arenaviruses.

Clinical presentation: Patients reported to date have presented with fever, headache, and myalgias. Within the first week, lymphopenia (25 to 700 per mm^3) and thrombocytopenia (30,000 to 40,000 per mm^3) were observed. Later complications included acute respiratory distress syndrome, liver failure, and hemorrhagic diatheses. Both of the reported patients died after 1 to 8 weeks.

Specimens for diagnostic testing: serum, liver, spleen, throat washings, body fluids

Patient isolation precautions: standard

Suggested assays for virus detection: detection of viral RNA by RT-PCR, virus isolation in cell cultures

Serodiagnosis: enzyme-linked immunosorbent assays for IgM and IgG antibodies, neutralization tests for confirmation

Biosafety level required for working with Whitewater Arroyo virus: BSL-3

Additional reading

Buchmeier MJ, Bowen MD, Peters CJ. Arenaviridae: the viruses and their replication. In: Knipe DM, Howley PM, editors. Fields virology. Vol 2. 4th ed. Philadelphia: Lippincott Williams & Wilkins; 2001. p. 1635–68.

Calisher CH, Nabity S, Root JJ, et al. Transmission of an arenavirus in white-throated woodrats (*Neotoma albigula*), southeastern Colorado. Emerg Infect Dis 2001;7:397–402.

Fulhorst CF, Bowen MD, Ksiazek TG, et al. Isolation and characterization of Whitewater Arroyo virus, a novel North American arenavirus. Virology 1996;224:114–20.

Fulhorst CF, Charrel RN, Weaver SC, et al. Geographic distribution and genetic diversity of Whitewater Arroyo virus in the southwestern United States. Emerg Infect Dis 2001;7:403–7.

Yellow fever

Agent: yellow fever virus, family Flaviviridae, genus *Flavivirus* (RNA)

Reservoir: humans, mosquitoes, monkeys, possibly ticks

Vector: mosquito (*Aedes*, *Haemagogus*, and *Sabethes* spp)

Vehicle: none

Incubation period: 3 d–6 d (range to 14 d)

Clinical hints:

backache	jaundice
headache	myalgias
hemorrhagic diathesis	relative bradycardia
illness is often biphasic	vomiting

Typical therapy: symptomatic

Disease distribution:

Angola	Ethiopia
Benin	French Guiana
Bolivia	Gabon
Brazil	Gambia
Burkina Faso	Ghana
Burundi	Guinea
Cameroon	Guinea Bissau
Central African Republic	Guyana
Chad	Ivory Coast
Colombia	Kenya
Congo	Liberia
Democratic Republic of Congo	Mali
	Mauritania
Ecuador	Niger
Equatorial Guinea	Nigeria

Panama	Suriname
Peru	Tanzania
Rwanda	Togo
Sao Tome and Principe	Uganda
Senegal	Venezuela
Sierra Leone	Zambia
Somalia	
Sudan	

Considered a potential bioterrorism weapon.

Notes

Transmission of yellow fever virus follows three patterns: sylvatic (or jungle), intermediate, and urban. The following definitions are extracted from WHO publications:

"Sylvatic yellow fever: In tropical rainforests, yellow fever occurs in monkeys that are infected via mosquitoes. The infected monkeys can then pass the virus onto other mosquitoes that feed on them. These infected mosquitoes bite humans entering the forest, resulting in sporadic cases of yellow fever. The majority of cases are young men working in the forest (logging, etc). On occasion, the virus spreads beyond the affected individual."

"Intermediate yellow fever: In humid or semi-humid savannas of Africa, small-scale epidemics occur. These behave differently from urban epidemics; many separate villages in an area suffer cases simultaneously, but fewer people are infected. Semi-domestic mosquitoes infect both monkey and human hosts. This area is often called the 'zone of emergence', where increased contact between humans and infected mosquitoes leads to disease. This is the most common type of outbreak seen in recent decades in Africa. It can shift to a more severe urban-type epidemic if the infection is carried into a suitable environment (with the presence of domestic mosquitoes and unvaccinated humans)."

"Urban yellow fever: Large epidemics can occur when migrants introduce the virus into areas with high population densities of unvaccinated humans. Domestic mosquitoes (*Aedes aegypti*) carry the virus from person to person; no monkeys are involved in transmission. These outbreaks tend to spread outwards from one source to cover a wide area."

Nigeria accounted for 90.8% of all yellow fever cases during 1989 to 1993. Peru accounted for 50% of all cases in 1995. In 1996, Senegal accounted for 30.2% of the world's cases, and Benin for 28.3%. In 1997, Bolivia accounted for 33.2% of the world's cases, and Peru for 23.2%. Peru accounted for 54.5% of cases in 1998.

Reports from Africa (Figure 9; number of cases and number of fatal cases not available for all years) and Latin America (Figure 10; fatal cases noted from 1971 only) indicate continual transmission at low level, with periodic epidemic transmission.

The last case of urban yellow fever in the Americas was reported in 1954.

Thirteen species of African mosquitoes are capable of transmitting yellow fever in the laboratory. The natural African vectors are *Aedes aegypti* (urban), *Aedes africanus* (jungle), *Aedes simpsoni*, and *Aedes furcifer-taylori*. *Ae. simpsoni* is found only in South Africa and Zimbabwe, and could theoretically transmit disease. *Aedes bromeliae* is a vector to both humans and monkeys in Central and Eastern Africa.

Ixodid ticks (*Amblyomma* spp) may serve as reservoirs in West Africa, and vertical transmission among culicine mosquitoes may allow virus survival in interepidemic periods.

Ae. aegypti was eradicated from most of South America during the first half of the 20th century, but reappeared during the

Yellow fever 217

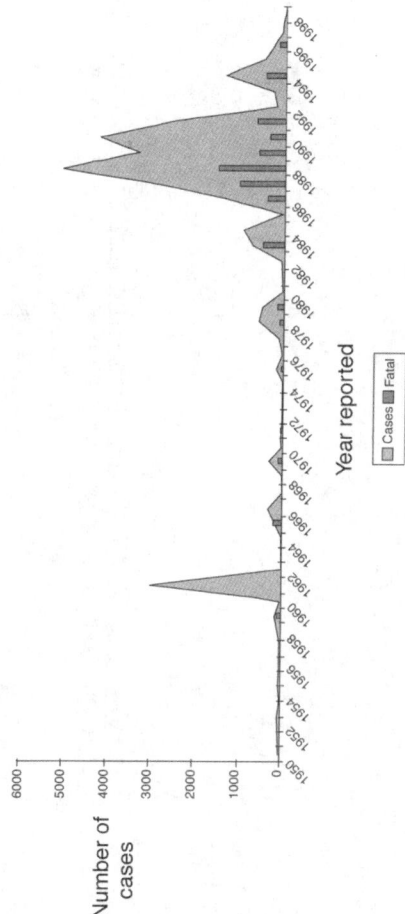

Figure 9 Yellow fever in Africa.

218 Exotic Viral Diseases

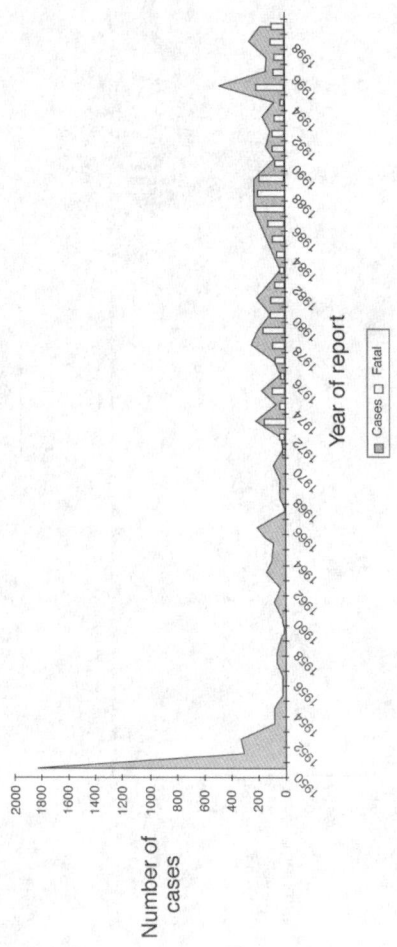

Figure 10 Yellow fever in Latin America.

1970s. Urban yellow fever had virtually disappeared from the continent, but was reported for the first time in Bolivia during 1997 to 1998, following a hiatus of 44 years. The American vectors are *Ae. aegypti*, *Haemagogus janthinomys*, *Haemagogus spegazzinii*, *Haemagogus leucocelaenus*, and *Sabethes chloropterus*. *Ae. aegypti* was eradicated from 21 countries in the American Region during 1948 to 1962; however, as of 1996, the mosquito is found in all countries in the area, except Bermuda, Canada, Chile, and Uruguay.

Clinical presentation: The clinical presentation of yellow fever can range from a self-limited flu-like illness to overwhelming hemorrhagic fever, with a case-fatality rate of 50%. As many as 50% of infections may be clinically inapparent. Infection is heralded by abrupt onset of fever, headache, and myalgias associated with conjunctival injection, facial flushing, relative bradycardia (Faget's sign), and leukopenia. Although most cases do not progress beyond this stage, remission of fever for a few hours to several days is followed by high fever, headache, lumbosacral pain, nausea, vomiting, abdominal pain, and somnolence. At this stage, the patient exhibits icteric hepatitis and a hemorrhagic diathesis with prominent bleeding from the gastrointestinal tract, epistaxis, bleeding gums, and petechial and purpuric hemorrhages. Weakness, prostration, protracted vomiting, and albuminuria are prominent. Deepening jaundice and elevations in serum transaminase levels continue for several days, accompanied by azotemia and progressive oliguria. Direct bilirubin levels rise to 5 to 10 mg/dL, whereas alkaline phosphatase levels are only slightly raised. Eventually, hypotension, shock, and metabolic acidosis develop, compounded by myocardial dysfunction and arrhythmias. Additional findings may include acute tubular necrosis, confusion, seizures, and coma. CSF examination reveals an elevated protein level without pleocytosis. Death usually occurs within 7 to 10 days after onset of the disease.

Specimens for diagnostic testing: blood, tissue (liver), serum

Patient isolation precautions: scrupulously avoid access by mosquitoes

Suggested assays for virus detection: detection of viral RNA by RT-PCR, virus isolation in cell cultures

Serodiagnosis: enzyme-linked immunosorbent assays for IgM and IgG antibodies, neutralization tests for confirmation

Biosafety level required for working with yellow fever virus: BSL-3

Additional reading

Anon. Advice for travelers. Med Lett Drugs Ther 1998;40:47–50.
Anon. Yellow fever. Wkly Epidemiol Rec 1998;73:351–2.
Barrett AD. Yellow fever vaccines. Biologicals 1997;25:17–25.
Jong EC. Travel immunizations. Med Clin North Am 1999;83:903–22.
Monath TP. Yellow fever: Victor, Victoria? Conqueror, conquest? Epidemics and research in the last forty years and prospects for the future. Am J Trop Med Hyg 1991;45:1–43.
http://www.who.int/emc/diseases/ebola/index.html (accessed September 21, 2002).
http://www.cdc.gov/ncidod/diseases/list_mosquitoborne.htm (accessed September 21, 2002).
http://www.cdc.gov/ncidod/dvbid/yellowfever/index.htm (accessed September 21, 2002).
http://www.emedicine.com/emerg/topic887.htm (accessed September 21, 2002).
http://www.emedicine.com/emerg/topic645.htm (accessed September 21, 2002).

Etiologic agents of exotic viral diseases

Alagoas virus
Alenquer virus
Alfuy virus
Alma-Arasan virus
Andes virus
Apeu virus
Apoi virus
Arboledas virus
Argentine hemorrhagic fever (Junin) virus
Banzi virus
Barmah Forest virus
Batai virus
Bayou virus
Belgrade virus
Bhanjavirus
Black Creek Canal virus
Bolivian hemorrhagic fever (Machupo) virus
Brazilian hemorrhagic fever (Sabia) virus
Buffalopox virus
Bujaru virus
Bunyamwera virus
Bunyaviruses (miscellaneous)
Bussuquara virus
Bwamba virus
Cacao virus
Cache Valley virus
California serogroup viruses
Calovo virus
Camelpox virus

Candiru virus
Cano Delgadito virus
Cantagalo virus
Caraparu virus
Catu virus
Cercopithecine herpesvirus
Chagres virus
Chandipura virus
Chikungunya virus
Choclo virus
Cocal virus
Colorado tick fever virus
Cowpox virus
Crimean-Congo hemorrhagic fever virus
Dengue viruses
Dhori virus
Dobrava virus
Dugbe virus
Eastern equine encephalitis virus
Ebola virus
Edge Hill virus
Erve virus
Everglades virus
Fakeeh virus
Fort Sherman virus
Gan Gan virus
Garissa virus
Germiston virus
Group C viruses
Guama virus
Guanarito (Venezuelan hemorrhagic fever) virus
Guaroa virus

Hantaan virus
Hantaviruses (New World)
Hantaviruses (Old World)
Hendra virus
Herpes virus B
Igbo Ora virus
Ilesha virus
Ilheus virus
Inkoo virus
Itaqui virus
Jamestown Canyon virus
Junin (Argentine hemorrhagic fever) virus
Juquitiba virus
Karshi virus
Keystone virus
Kokobera virus
Koutango virus
Kunjin virus
Kyasanur Forest disease virus
La Crosse virus
Laguna Negra virus
Langat virus
Lassa virus
Louping ill virus
Lumbo virus
Lymphocytic choriomeningitis virus
Machupo (Bolivian hemorrhagic fever) virus
Madrid virus
Marburg virus
Marituba virus
Mayaro virus
Me Tri virus

Meaban virus
Menangle virus
Modoc virus
Monkeypox virus
Monongahela virus
Murray Valley encephalitis virus
Murutucu virus
Nairobi sheep disease virus
Negishi virus
New World phleboviruses
New York-1 virus
Ngari virus
Nipah virus
Northway virus
Nyando virus
Ockelbo virus
Omsk hemorrhagic fever virus
O'nyong-nyong virus
Oran virus
Orf virus
Oriboca virus
Oropouche virus
Ossa virus
Piry virus
Pirital virus
Pogosta virus
Pongola virus
Powassan virus
Pseudocowpox virus
Punta Toro virus
Puumala virus
Restan virus

Etiologic agents of exotic viral diseases 225

Rift Valley fever virus
Rio Bravo virus
Rocio virus
Ross River virus
Sabia (Brazilian hemorrhagic fever) virus
Sandfly fever Naples virus
Sandfly fever Sicilian virus
Semliki Forest virus
Seoul virus
Sepik virus
Shokwe virus
Simbu group viruses
Sin Nombre virus
Sindbis virus
Snowshoe hare virus
Spondweni virus
St. Louis encephalitis virus
Stratford virus
Tacaiuma virus
Tahyna virus
Tamdy virus
Tanapox virus
Tensaw virus
Thogoto virus
Tick-borne encephalitis virus (Central European)
Tick-borne encephalitis virus (Russian spring-summer)
Tonate virus
Toscana virus
Tribec virus
Trivittatus virus
Trubanaman virus
Tyuleniy virus

Usutu virus
Vaccinia virus
Venezuelan equine encephalitis virus
Venezuelan hemorrhagic fever (Guanarito) virus
Vesicular stomatitis Indiana virus
Vesicular stomatitis New Jersey virus
Wanowrie virus
Wesselsbron virus
West Nile virus
Western equine encephalitis virus
Whitewater Arroyo virus
Wyeomyia virus
Yellow fever virus
Zika virus

Appendix A
Sample collection, shipment, and testing

Rapid and specific, or provisional, identification of the etiologic agent of an exotic viral illness can lead to suitable treatment of the patient, and simultaneously allow public health authorities to take measures intended to prevent community outbreaks or epidemics. Whole blood and serum, taken for virus isolation attempts, should be processed immediately or placed on dry ice (−70°C), or otherwise suitably frozen until they can be tested at a local, state, national, commercial, or other laboratory. Although not a critical issue for antigen detection, specimens for testing should be shipped and stored at low temperatures to prevent further degradation of proteins and nucleic acids. When sera are to be tested for antibody only, they can be shipped and stored at ambient temperatures, unless they are contaminated with microorganisms or will be in transit for long periods or exposed to high temperatures.

Special safety precautions are recommended for many viruses, and work with specimens that might contain these viruses is best left to those who have relevant experience and suitable, secure working facilities. Should a patient present with signs and symptoms of infection that can be highly linked to any of these exotic viruses, local or national health departments should be notified at once. These organizations will make further determinations and provide information relative to containment as well as contact with laboratories having high security facilities.

Specimens suggested for the diagnosis of specific infections

Blood (not frozen): Chikungunya, Colorado tick fever, Ebola, Ilheus, Bussuquara, Kyasanur Forest disease, louping ill, Marburg, Mayaro, Old World sandfly fevers, Omsk hemorrhagic fever, O'nyong-nyong, Oropouche, Rift Valley fever, Sindbis, Spondweni, Thogoto, tick-borne encephalitis (Central European), tick-borne encephalitis (Russian spring-summer), vesicular stomatitis, Wesselsbron, West Nile, and yellow fever viruses

CSF: California serogroup virus, Crimean-Congo hemorrhagic fever, eastern equine encephalitis, Japanese encephalitis, louping ill, lymphocytic choriomeningitis, Murray Valley encephalitis, Nipah, Oropouche, Powassan, Rift Valley fever, St. Louis encephalitis, Thogoto, tick-borne encephalitis (Central European), tick-borne encephalitis (Russian spring-summer), Venezuelan equine encephalitis, western equine encephalitis, and West Nile

Serum (acute-phase and, if possible, convalescent-phase): all diseases

Tissue and body fluids

Brain: eastern equine encephalitis, Japanese encephalitis, Murray Valley encephalitis, Nipah, Rocio, St. Louis encephalitis, Thogoto, tick-borne encephalitis (Central European), tick-borne encephalitis (Russian spring-summer), Venezuelan equine encephalitis, western equine encephalitis viruses

Various: Crimean-Congo hemorrhagic fever, dengue and Whitewater Arroyo viruses

Liver: Argentine hemorrhagic fever, Bolivian hemorrhagic fever, Brazilian hemorrhagic fever, Ebola, Lassa, Marburg, Venezuelan hemorrhagic fever, Whitewater Arroyo, and yellow fever viruses

Spleen: Argentine hemorrhagic fever, Bolivian hemorrhagic fever, Brazilian hemorrhagic fever, Ebola, Lassa, Marburg, Venezuelan hemorrhagic fever and Whitewater Arroyo viruses

Skin tissue or exudate: cowpox, herpes virus B, monkeypox, Orf virus, pseudocowpox, Sindbis, and tanapox viruses

Throat swab or washings: Lassa, lymphocytic choriomeningitis, Venezuelan equine encephalitis, Wesselsbron disease, Whitewater Arroyo viruses

Appendix B
Diagnostic tests

Virus isolation, viral antigen detection, electron microscopy, and other methods have been used to determine the etiologic agents of viral diseases. However, the most rapid and specific detection of a virus is by the rapidly advancing field of molecular technology, such as reverse transcription-polymerase chain reaction (RT-PCR). RT-PCR is also useful for molecular epidemiologic and evolutionary analyses, so that the origin of the virus can be ascertained. This method does not provide an isolate with which to determine phenotypic characteristics of the virus.

Serologically **confirmed** infection with a virus requires demonstration of at least a fourfold increase or decrease in antibody titer between paired acute-phase and convalescent-phase serum samples, collected days to weeks or months apart. A serologically **presumptive** infection is one in which only an acute-phase serum is available, but which contains IgM (acute) antibody to the virus, and for which other assays show high titer to the virus, including those for IgG antibody. Often, the collection and testing of another serum sample later in the illness reveals antibody of sufficient titer to allow the designation to be shifted from "presumptive" to "confirmed." A definition of **inconclusive** is a temporizing one, indicating that only an acute-phase sample is available, one which contains no IgM antibody, and is negative or has a very low titer to the virus by other assay methods. Any other results should be considered **negative**. The assays that can be used include neutralization, enzyme-linked immunosorbent assay (ELISA) for IgM or IgG antibody, and immunofluorescence, among others.

Recommended diagnostic assay(s): For virus detection, either RT-PCR or virus isolation can be used, although the former is usually more rapidly accomplished. For serodiagnosis, paired (acute- and convalescent-phase) serum samples should be tested by ELISA for IgM and IgG antibodies. Adjunct or alternative tests include hemagglutination-inhibition, complement-fixation, and immunofluorescence. Neutralization tests are the *sine qua non* of serodiagnostic confirmation.

Reasons for use of these assays: Having a virus isolate or detecting its nucleic acid is the only definitive way to determine the presence of a particular virus in a patient. Therefore, the above-mentioned assays are the methods of choice. Neutralization tests provide the most specific evidence for infection with a specific virus and the greatest degree of confidence when conducting serodiagnosis. However, neutralization tests require specialized containment facilities, laboratory personnel having expertise in safe handling of viruses, and live viruses, as well as cell cultures, media, and specialized personnel to care for them and to interpret the results.

IgG antibody is usually detectable within a few days after onset of the viral illness. Therefore, detection of the IgG antibody by ELISA can be taken to indicate evidence of infection with a virus, but it cannot be used to determine whether that infection was recent or remote. If adequately paired samples are available, dynamic changes in IgG antibody titer to a virus are considered to be conclusive evidence for recent infection with that virus or a closely-related one.

IgM antibody, also determined by ELISA, is a "first-responder" in virus infections, and its presence is taken to indicate a recent infection. Thus, the presence of IgM antibody to a virus in a single sample is considered at least provisional, at most presumptive, evidence for infection with that specific virus or a closely-related one. However, IgM antibody may persist for 30 to 90 days or longer (perhaps for years) in certain individuals, and therefore its presence in a single serum cannot be used to provide conclusive evidence for infection with that virus. Nonetheless, if adequately paired samples are available, dynamic changes in IgM antibody titer to a virus are considered conclusive evidence for recent infection with that virus, or a closely-related virus.

Many of the various serologic assays that have been used, such as hemagglutination-inhibition, complement-fixation, and immunofluorescence, were developed in the earlier days of the field of virology. The hemagglutination-inhibition (HI) assay measures the capacity of a serum or cerebrospinal fluid to prevent a viral antigen (hemagglutinin) from forming "bridges" between erythrocytes of appropriate species. Because viral hemagglutinins generally are viral surface (or envelope) proteins, and because these surface proteins are shared by many viruses within particular groups of viruses, the HI test may measure antibody to any of many viruses. For example, HI antibody to St. Louis encephalitis virus will react not only with antigen of St. Louis encephalitis virus, but with antigen of West Nile virus, Japanese encephalitis, Murray Valley encephalitis, and other flaviviruses as well. The extent to which reactivity occurs, as measured by the antibody titer of the serum, depends on the antigenic relationships of these viruses; that is, antibody to viruses more closely related to one another react to higher titer than does antibody to viruses that are less closely related. Thus, HI antibody in a patient can be used to determine at least the serogroup of the infecting virus, but it cannot be used to determine the specific virus.

In the complement-fixation (CF) assay, complement-fixing antibody is directed against viral nucleocapsid, which comprises antigens that may be relatively type-specific, antigenic complex-specific, or group-specific, depending on the virus.

Assays for CF antibody can provide relatively specific results, for example, in determining which of the dengue viruses caused an infection. However, because CF antibody can only be detected many days after onset, is a relatively complex assay, and is not particularly sensitive in detecting antibody, it has fallen out of favor in modern use. Moreover, CF antibody is essentially always IgG antibody, so it does not provide diagnostic clues regarding very recent infections.

As are CF antibody assays, immunofluorescence (IF) assays are less type-specific than they are group- or complex-specific. However, IF assays can be configured to detect either IgM or IgG antibody, and are relatively simple to conduct.

Many other assays, including radioimmunoassays, time-resolved fluoroimmunoassays, immunodiffusion, and reverse passive hemagglutination, have been used. Some of these hold advantages over others, but all have their disadvantages, as do all antibody assays. In addition to complexity of performance, the collective reasons of cost, specificity, lack of sufficient training of laboratory workers, and in particular, the need for adequate and expert interpretation, have caused these tests to be less frequently used. This is not to say that antibody assays in current vogue are used because they are simple and inexpensive to perform. Tests such as ELISA have superceded other assays, because standardization of ELISA protocols provides simplicity of performance and uniformity of required reagents. In addition, and more important insofar as the patient and community are concerned, ELISA is sensitive and no less specific in detecting IgG antibody. Indeed, ELISA, in the form of IgM antibody capture assays, is the test of choice for detecting IgM antibody. No matter which of these tests is used, the neutralization test is the definitive assay because it is the most specific, and it provides information regarding the immune status of the patient as well.

Anticipated results: Depending on the interval between infection and day of collection, on the characteristics of the infection of any given patient, on the preservation of the sample, and on other variables, the probability of virus isolation may not be high. Detection of viral nucleic acid by RT-PCR provides a greater probability of success, because that nucleic acid may persist in the patient long after infectious virus can be isolated.

IgM antibody should be detectable on or within a day or two of onset of illness, and IgG antibody within a day or two of that. In all cases, where possible, neutralization tests should be done by a recognized reference center, one which can include tests for antibody to the suspected agent as well as for other related viruses.

Hemagglutination-inhibition, complement-fixation, and immunofluorescence, detect both IgM and IgG antibodies and can provide adequate evidence for the presence of antibody to a virus, particularly when paired samples are available. All these tests can be either very broadly cross-reactive or of narrow specificity, depending on the infecting virus. Therefore, although appropriate, they may not always provide definitive results.

Additional reading

Knipe DM, Howley PM, editors. Fields virology. 4th ed. Philadelphia: Lippincott Williams & Wilkins; 2001.

Lennette EH, Smith TF, editors. Laboratory diagnosis of viral infections. 3rd ed. New York: Marcel Dekker, Inc; 1999.

Service MW, editor. The encyclopedia of arthropod-transmitted infections. New York: CABI Publishing; 2001.

Appendix C
Drugs and Vaccines

Drugs

Although a number of drugs are used in the treatment of viral hepatitis, varicella, cytomegalovirus, AIDS, and other viral infections, only two agents are available for diseases discussed in this text: Acyclovir, used for herpes virus B infection; and Ribavirin, used for arenaviruses, Old-World hantaviruses, and Crimean-Congo hemorrhagic fever virus. These two drugs are summarized below.

Acyclovir

Mechanism of action: a synthetic guanine analogue, which is converted by viral kinases to a triphosphate which then inhibits incorporation of DNA-polymerase into DNA

Dosage: see herpevirus B virus infection

CSF penetration (inflamed meninges): 50% of serum level

Typical drug dosing for renal dysfunction: dosage interval should be extended to twice daily if creatinine clearance is less than 50 mL/min, and once daily if creatinine clearance is less than 10 mL/min; an additional dose need not be given following hemodialysis; the dosage is not altered by continuous peritoneal dialysis

Potential toxic effects:

arthalgia or arthritis

confusion

delusions

depression

diarrhea

encephalitis or encephalopathy

fever
hallucinations
headache
hepatic dysfunction / hepatitis
insomnia
lymphadenopathy
nausea / vomiting
paresthesia
psychosis
rash
renal toxicity / dysfunction
seizures
somnolence
thrombocytosis
urolithiasis
vertigo or dizziness
visual disturbance

Drug interactions:

Aminoglycosides – may increase risk for nephro/ototoxicity with Acyclovir
Cimetidine – interacts (details not given) with Acyclovir
Foscarnet – risk for nephro/ototoxicity with Acyclovir
Opiate – levels are decreased by Acyclovir
Probenecid – reduces the excretion of Acyclovir
Zidovidine – causes lethargy in combination with Acyclovir

Proprietary names:

Aciciclin
Aciclobeta
Aciclosina
Aciclostad
Aci-Sanorania
Aciviran

Activir
Acycloftal
Acyclo-V
Acyvir
Alovir
Aviral
Avirase
Avix
Avyclor
Avyplus
Ceviran
Cicloviral
Citivir
Clonorax
Clovix
Cusiviral
Cyclivex
Cycloviran
Divicil
Dravir
Efriviral
Esavir
Geavir
Hermixofex
Hermocil
Herpetad
Herpofug
Herpoviric
Maynor
Milavir
Neviran
Orivir
Rexan

Sifiviral
Viclovir
Vipral
Virasorb
Virberpes
Virmen
Viropos
Virovir
Viruseen
Zoliparin
Zoviplus
Zovir
Zovirax

Drug spectrum:

Herpes simplex virus
Herpes virus B
Varicella-Zoster virus

Ribavirin

Mechanism of action: a synthetic guanine analogue which acts on messenger RNA and nucleotide metabolism (production of guanosine triphosphate pools)

Dosage: see specific diseases

CSF penetration (inflamed meninges): 67 to >100% of serum level

Typical drug dosing for renal dysfunction: no adjustment is necessary for patients with reduced creatinine clearance, or during hemodialysis or continuous peritoneal dialysis.

Potential toxic effects:

anemia
conjunctivitis

headache
hemolysis
insomnia
nausea / vomiting
pregnancy (contraindicated)
rash
somnolence

Drug interactions:

Clarithromycin – interacts (details not given) with Ribavirin
Zalcitabine (ddC) – increases risk for neurotoxicity from Ribavirin
Zidovidine – activity is increased by Ribavirin

Proprietary names:

Rebetol
Tribavirin
Virazole

Drug spectrum:

Argentine hemorrhagic fever
Bolivian hemorrhagic fever
Crimean-Congo hemorrhagic fever
Hantaviruses (Old World)
Lassa fever
Brazilian hemorrhagic fever

Vaccines

Commercial vaccines are available for prevention of Argentine hemorrhagic fever, Old World Hantaviruses, tick-borne encephalitis, and yellow fever. An immune globulin preparation is available to protect against tick-borne encephalitis. This preparation is not recommended for use because concerns about enhancement of infections, and is not widely available.

Argentine hemorrhagic fever

Content: live attenuated Junin virus strain XJ; 40,000 pfu/mL

Typical adult dosage: 1.0 mL IM (deltoid)

Typical pediatric dosage: not established

Subsequent booster: not established

Toxic effects:

arthralgia / arthritis
headache
myalgia
nausea or vomiting

Contraindications:

allergy to the vaccine
concurrent tacrolimus
immune deficiency (live-agent preparations)
pregnancy

Proprietary name:

Candid 1

Hantavirus (Old World)

Content: formalin-inactivated Hantaan virus ROK 84-105 from suckling mouse brain, 10,240 ELISA units/mL

Typical adult dosage: 0.5 mL IM at 0 and 30 days

Typical pediatric dosage: unknown

Subsequent booster: 0.5 mL at 12 months

Toxic effects: nausea or vomiting

Contraindications: none

Proprietary name: Hantavax (available in South Korea)

Tick-borne encephalitis

Content: inactivated virus for use in endemic areas, prepared from tick strain passed through mouse brain and chicken embryo cells

Typical adult dosage: 0.5 mL IM at 0, 1 to 3, and 9 to 12 months

Typical pediatric dosage: age 1 year or more, dosages as for adult

Subsequent booster: single booster after 3 to 6 years

Toxic effects:

fever
headache
lymphadenopathy
nausea or vomiting
neuropathy
rash (various forms)

Contraindications:

allergy (sensitivity) to thimerosal
allergy to eggs
allergy to the vaccine

Proprietary names:

Encepur
FSME-Immun
Tico Vac

Tick-borne encephalitis globulin

Content: immunoglobulin concentrate (titer at least 640)

Typical adult dosage: preexposure, 0.05 mL/kg IM; postexposure, 0.2 mL/kg IM within 96 h of exposure

Typical pediatric dosage: contraindicated below age 14 due to concerns over enhancement of infection

Subsequent booster: every 4 weeks if necessary

Toxic effects: none

Contraindications:

defer live measles (etc) vaccine for >3 months

Proprietary names:
Encegam
FSME-bulin

Japanese encephalitis

Content: inactivated (mouse brain or hamster kidney) or attenuated (hamster kidney) virus

Typical adult dosage: 1.0 mL SQ days 0, 7, 14 to 30, indicated for those anticipating residence or extended travel to endemic areas

Typical pediatric dosage: ages 1 to 3 years, 0.5 mL SQ on days 0, 7, 14 to 30; over 3 years, 1.0 mL SQ on days 0, 7, 14 to 30

Subsequent booster: after 3 years

Toxic effects:

abdominal pain
encephalitis (encephalopathy)
erythema multiforme
fever
Guillain-Barre syndrome
headache
myalgia
nausea or vomiting
neuropathy

rash (various forms)
seizures

Contraindications:

allergy (sensitivity) to thimerosal
allergy to the vaccine
concurrent severe acute illness
immune deficiency (live-agent preparations)

Proprietary name: JE-Vax

Yellow fever

Content: live attenuated 17D strain derived from fertilized hens' eggs

Typical adult dosage: 0.5 mL SQ

Typical pediatric dosage: minimum age 9 months, 0.5 mL SQ

Subsequent booster: every 10 years

Toxic effects:

encephalitis (encephalopathy)
fever
headache
infection by vaccine virus (rare)
lymphadenopathy
myalgia
nausea or vomiting
seizures

Contraindications:

allergy to eggs
allergy to the vaccine
concurrent tacrolimus
defer cholera vaccine for > 3 weeks

immune deficiency (live-agent preparations)
pregnancy

Proprietary names:

Amaril
Arilax
Stamaril
YF-Vax

Index

In this index, page numbers followed by the letter "t" designate tables. *See also* cross references designate related topics or more detailed subtopic listings.

A

Acute epidemic hemorrhagic fever, 89–94
Acute infectious capillary toxinosis, 58–63
Acyclovir, 235–239
  drug interactions with, 236
  Herpes virus B, 98
Aerosol
  viral transmission route, 12t
African green monkey disease, 119–121
AHF, 22–25, 240
Alenquer virus, 132
Alfuy virus, 28
Alkhurma virus, 107–108
Alma-Arasan, 187
Alphavirus, 164
Amaril
  Japanese encephalitis, 244
American mountain fever, 52–54
Aminoglycosides
  interactions with acyclovir, 236
Andes virus, 86
Animal bite
  virus transmitted, 11t
Animal contact
  viral transmission route, 12t
Apeu, 80
Apoi virus, 104
Arboledas virus, 132
Argentine hemorrhagic fever (AHF), 22–25, 240
Arilax
  Japanese encephalitis, 244

Arthralgia
  differential diagnosis, 17t
Arthritis
  differential diagnosis, 17t
Australian encephalitis, 128–131
Australian X disease, 128–131

B

Banzi virus, 171
Barmah Forest *(Alphavirus),* 164
Barmah Forest virus disease (BFD), 26–30
Bat
  natural reservoirs, 13t
Batai virus, 39
Bat paramyxovirus, 95–97
Bayou virus, 86
Bermejo virus, 86
BFD, 26–30
Bhanja virus, 38
BHF, 24, 31–33
Bird
  natural reservoirs, 13t
Black Creek Canal virus, 85
Blood, 227–228
Body fluids, 228
Bolivian hemorrhagic fever (BHF), 24, 31–33
Bosnian hemorrhagic fever, 89–94
Bouquet fever, 64–70
Brazilian hemorrhagic fever, 34–35
Break-bone fever, 64–70
Buffalopox, 56

Bujaru virus, 132
Bunyamwera virus, 38
Bunyavirus infections, 36–42
Bussuquara fever, 101–102
Bwamba virus, 36, 38

C

Cacao virus, 132
Calabazo virus, 86
California serogroup, 38
California serogroup virus
　　　　infections, 43–47
Calovo virus, 39
Camelpox, 55
Candid 1, 240
Candiru virus, 132
Cano Delgadito virus, 86
Cantagalo virus, 56
Caraparu, 80
Cat
　natural reservoirs, 14t
Cattle
　natural reservoirs, 14t
Catu virus, 39, 80
CCHF, 58–63
Centers for Disease Control and
　　　　Prevention (CDC), 5
Cercopithecine herpesvirus 1
　　　　infection, 98–100
CF assay, 232–233
Chagres virus, 132
Chandipura, 197
Changuinola virus, 132
Chikungunya virus infection,
　　　　48–51
Choclo virus, 86
Churilov disease, 89–94
Cimetidine
　interactions with acyclovir,
　　　　236
Clarithromycin
　interactions with Ribavirin, 239

Clinical history
　exotic viral infection, 6
Colorado tick fever (CTF), 52–54
Complement-fixation (CF) assay,
　　　　232–233
Conjunctivitis
　differential diagnosis, 17t–18t
Contagious pustular dermatitis,
　　　　146–147
Convict Creek virus, 85
Cowpox disease, 55–57
Crimean-Congo hemorrhagic
　　　　fever (CCHF), 58–63
CSF, 228

D

Dairy products
　viral transmission route, 12t
Dandy fever, 64–70
Date fever, 64–70
ddC
　interactions with Ribavirin, 239
Deer
　natural reservoirs, 14t
Definitive diagnosis, 6
Dengue fever (DF), 64–70
Dengue hemorrhagic fever (DHF),
　　　　66–89
DF, 64–70
DHF, 66–89
Dhori virus, 179
Diagnosis
　rapid
　　importance of, 3
Diagnostic assays, 230–231
Diagnostic tests, 230–234
Differential diagnosis, 17t–21t
Dobrava-Belgrade virus, 91
Dobrava-Belgrade virus infection,
　　　　89–94
Droplets
　viral transmission route, 12t

Drug interactions
  with acyclovir, 236
  with Ribavirin, 239
Drugs, 235–244. *See also* individual names
Duengero, 64–70
Dugbe virus, 60
Durba syndrome, 119–121
Dust
  viral transmission route, 12t

E

Eastern equine encephalitis (EEE), 71–75
Ebola hemorrhagic fever, 76–79
Ecthyma contagiosum, 146–147
Edge Hill *(Flavivirus),* 164
Edge Hill virus, 28
EEE, 71–75
Electronic information networks, 5
Encegam, 242
Encephalitis
  differential diagnosis, 18t–19t
Encepur, 241–244
Endemic benign nephropathy, 89–94
Enzootic hepatitis, 156–159
Epidemic hemorrhagic fever, 89–94
Equine morbillivirus, 95–97
Erve virus, 59
Etiologic agents, 221–226
European tick-borne encephalitis, 182–185
Everglades virus (VEE II), 190
Exposure history, 5

F

Fakeeh virus, 107
Far Eastern encephalitis, 183
Far Eastern hemorrhagic fever, 89–94

Far Eastern tick-borne encephalitis, 186–188
Fever with rash
  differential diagnosis, 20t
Flavivirus, 164
Fort Sherman virus, 39
Foscarnet
  interactions with acyclovir, 236
FSME-bulin, 242
FSME-Immun, 241

G

Gancyclovir
  Herpes virus B, 98
Gandy fever, 64–70
Ganjam virus, 60
Garissa virus, 38
Geographic medicine, 5
Germiston virus, 38
GIDEON, 5
Giraffe fever, 64–70
Group C viral fevers, 80–83
Group C virus, 38
Guama virus, 39, 81

H

Hantaan (HTN) virus, 91, 93
Hantavax, 240
Hantavirus infections (New World), 83–88
Hantavirus infections (Old World), 89–94, 240–241
Hantavirus pulmonary syndrome, 83–88
Hanzalova virus disease, 182–185
Hare
  natural reservoirs, 15t
Health Canada, 5
Hemagglutination-inhibition (HI) assay, 232
Hemorrhagic fever
  differential diagnosis, 19t

Hemorrhagic fever with renal syndrome (HFRS), 89–94
Hemorrhagic nephrosonephritis, 89–94
Hendra disease, 95–97
Herpes simiae virus infection, 98–100
Herpes virus B infection, 98–100
HFRS, 89–94
HI assay, 232
Horse
 natural reservoirs, 14t
HTN virus, 91, 93
Hu-39694 virus, 86
Hypr virus disease, 182–185

I

IF assays, 233
Igbo Ora virus, 144
IgG antibody
 detection of, 231
IgM antibody
 ELISA, 231
Ilesha virus, 38
Ilheus fever, 101–102
Immunization history, 5
Immunodiffusion, 233
Immunofluorescence, 232
Immunofluorescence (IF) assays, 233
Inconclusive
 definition, 230
Incubation period
 and travelers arrival and departure dates, 4
Infectious hemorrhagic fever, 89–94
Inkoo virus, 44
Intermediate yellow fever, 215–216
Itaqui, 81

J

Japanese encephalitis, 103–106, 242–243

JE-Vax, 243
Junin hemorrhagic fever, 22–25
Juquitiba virus, 86

K

Kangaroos. *See* Macropods
Karelian fever, 166
Karshi virus, 187
Keystone virus, 44
Khabarovsk disease, 89–94
Kinjiang hemorrhagic fever, 58–63
Kokobera virus, 28
Korean hemorrhagic fever, 89–94
Koutango virus, 171
Kumlinge virus disease, 182–185
Kyasanur Forest disease, 107–109

L

La Crosse encephalitis, 43
Lagomorph
 natural reservoirs, 15t
Laguna Negra virus, 86
Langat virus, 104
Lassa fever, 110–113
La tremblante du mouton, 114–115
Lechiguanas, 86
Liver, 228
Louping ill, 114–115
Lourdige, 202–207
Lumbo virus, 39
Lymphocytic choriomeningitis, 116–118

M

Machupo hemorrhagic fever, 31–33
Machupo virus, 32
Macropods
 natural reservoirs, 14t–15t
Madrid, 81

Marburg virus disease, 119–121
Marsupial
  natural reservoirs, 14t–15t
Mayaro fever, 122–124
Meaban virus, 187
Menalngle virus, 95–97
Meningitis
  differential diagnosis, 18t–19t
Me Tri virus, 49
Midge
  virus transmitted, 11t
Milker's nodule, 154–155
Modoc virus, 175
Monkey fever, 107–109
Monkeypox disease, 125–127
Monongahela virus, 86
Mosquito
  virus transmitted, 10t
Mountain fever, 52–54
Mountain tick fever, 52–54
Muroid virus nephropathy, 89–94
Murray Valley encephalitis, 128–131
Murutucu, 81
Muskrat fever, 140–142

N

Nairobi sheep disease, 59
Naples sandfly fever, 137–139
Naples virus, 138
Natural reservoirs, 13t–16t
Near Eastern equine encephalitis, 202–207
Negishi virus, 186
Nephropathia epidemica, 89–94
Neudoerfl virus disease, 182–185
Neutralization tests, 231
New World sandfly fevers, 132–133
New York -1 virus, 85
Ngari virus, 38
Nipah virus disease, 134–136

Northway virus, 40
Nyando virus, 39

O

Ockelbo disease, 166
Old World sandfly fevers, 137–139
Omsk hemorrhagic fever, 140–142
O'nyong-nyong, 143–145
Opiate
  interactions with acyclovir, 236
Oral secretions
  virus transmitted, 11t
Oran, 86
Orf, 146–147
Oropouche fever, 148–150
Oropouche virus, 38
Ossa, 81
Ostroff, Steven, 3
Ovine encephalomyelitis, 114–115
Ovine pustular dermatitis, 146–147

P

Pappataci fever, 137–139
Paramyxovirus, 95–97
Patient approach, 3
Peste loca, 189–192
Phiebotomus fever, 137–139
Phlebovirus, 38
Photophobia
  differential diagnosis, 17t–18t
Pirital virus, 193
Piry, 197
Pneumonia
  differential diagnosis, 21t
Pogosta disease, 166
Polka fever, 64–70
Pongola virus, 39
Powassan encephalitis, 151–153
Prevention, 8

Primate (nonhuman)
  natural reservoirs, 15t
Probenecid
  interactions with acyclovir, 236
ProMed, 5
Pseudocowpox, 154–155
Pulmonary failure
  differential diagnosis, 21t
Punta Toro virus, 132
Puumala (PUU) virus, 91, 93

R

Rabbit
  natural reservoirs, 15t
Radioimmunoassays, 233
Rebetol
  interactions with Ribavirin, 239
Renal dysfunction
  drug dosing for, 235–238
Reservoir
  defined, 2
Restan, 81
Reston strain, 77
Reverse passive hemagglutination, 233
Reverse transcription-polymerase chain reaction (RT-PCR), 6
Ribavirin, 7, 238–244
  AHF, 22
  BHF, 31
  CCHF, 58
  drug interactions with, 239
  Hendra virus, 95
  sabia, 34
Rift Valley fever, 156–159
Rio Bravo virus, 175
Rio Mamore virus, 86
Rocio encephalitis, 160–161
Rodent-borne viral nephropathy, 89–94
Rodents, 5
  natural reservoirs, 15t–16t

Ross River disease, 162–165
RT-PCR, 6
Russian autumnal encephalitis, 103–106
Russian spring-summer encephalitis virus, 183

S

Sabia, 34–35
Saddle-back fever, 6
Sample collection, 227–229
Scandinavian epidemic nephropathy, 89–94
Scottish sheep encephalomyelitis, 114–115
Seoul virus, 91
Sepik virus, 171
Serologically confirmed infection, 230
Serologically presumptive infection, 230
Serum, 228
Sheep
  natural reservoirs, 16t
Shipment, 227–229
Shokwe virus, 39
Sicilian sandfly fevers, 137–139
Sicilian virus, 138
Sindbis fever, 166–169
Sin Nombre virus, 85
Skin exudate, 229
Skin tissue, 229
Snowshoe hare virus, 44
Songo fever, 89–94
Specimens
  for diagnosis, 227–228
Spleen, 228
Spondweni fever, 170–172
Spring-Autumn fever, 140–142
St. Louis encephalitis, 173–176
Stamaril
  Japanese encephalitis, 244

Stratford *(Flavivirus)*, 164
Stratford virus, 28
Summer encephalitis, 103–106
Swine
    natural reservoirs, 15t
Sylvatic yellow fever, 215
Symptoms, 17t–21t
Syndromes, 17t–21t

T

Tacaiuma virus, 39
Tahyna virus, 44
Tanapox virus disease, 177–178
Tamdy virus, 39
Tensaw virus, 39
Testing, 227–229
Thogoto virus disease, 179–181
Throat swab, 229
Throat washings, 229
Thwarter ill, 114–115
Tick
    virus transmitted, 10t–11t
Tick-borne encephalitis, 241
Tick-borne encephalitis (Central European), 182–185
Tick-borne encephalitis globulin, 241–244
Tick-borne encephalitis (Russian spring-summer), 186–188
Tico Vac, 241
Time-resolved fluoroimmunoassays, 233
Tissue, 228
Tonate virus (VEE type IIIB), 190
Topografov disease, 89–94
Toscana virus, 138
Travelers
    arrival and departure dates of, 4
Trembling ill, 114–115
Tribavirin
    interactions with Ribavirin, 239
Tribee virus, 60

Trivittatus virus, 44
Trubanaman and Gan Gan viruses, 28
Tyuleniy virus, 187

U

Urban yellow fever, 216
Usutu virus, 171

V

Vaccines, 235–244, 239–240
Vaccinia, 55–57
Vectors, 10t–11t
    defined, 2
VEE, 73, 189–192
VEE II, 190
VEE type IIIB, 190
Vehicle
    defined, 2
Venezuelan equine encephalitis (VEE), 73, 189–192
Venezuelan hemorrhagic fever (VHF), 193–195
Vesciular/pustular enanthem or rash
    differential diagnosis, 20t–21t
Vesicular stomatitis, 196–198
Vesicular stomatitis Alagoas and Cocal, 197
Vesicular stomatitis Indiana, 197
Vesicular stomatitis New Jersey, 197
VHF, 193–195
Viral hemorrhagic fever, 89–94
Viral transmission
    routes of, 12t
Virazole
    interactions with Ribavirin, 239
Virus, 39

W

Wallaby. *See* Macropods

Wanowrile virus, 39
Wesselsbron disease, 199–201
Western equine encephalitis, 73, 208–210
West Nile virus encephalitis, 202–207
West Nile virus fever, 202–207
Whitewater Arroyo virus infection, 211–213
World Health Organization (WHO), 5
Wyeomyia virus, 39

Y
Yellow fever, 214–220

YF-Vax
    Japanese encephalitis, 244

Z
Zalcitabine
    interactions with Ribavirin, 239
Zidovidine
    interactions with acyclovir, 236
    interactions with Ribavirin, 239
Zika virus, 170
Zinga, 156–159